The Brain Food Diet for Children

THE BRAIN FOOD DIET FOR CHILDREN

*How to Improve Your Child's Intelligence
Through Proper Nutrition*

by
RALPH E. MINEAR, M.D., M.P.H.
Faculty Member, Harvard Medical School
Staff Pediatrician, Massachusetts General Hospital
with

William Proctor

THE BOBBS-MERRILL COMPANY, INC.
Indianapolis/New York

Published by The Bobbs-Merrill Co., Inc.
Indianapolis/New York
Manufactured in the United States of America
First Printing
Designed by Jacques Chazaud

Library of Congress Cataloging in Publication Data

Minear, Ralph E.
  The brain food diet for children.

  Includes index.
  1. Children—Nutrition.   2. Intellect—Nutritional aspects.   I. Proc-
tor, William. II. Title.
RJ206.M694 1983   649'.3   83-3798
ISBN 0-672-52755-3

ACKNOWLEDGMENTS

We are deeply grateful to those whose hard work has contributed to the final form of this manuscript.

First of all, we want to thank Dan Williams, whose outstanding research abilities and writing skills helped us pull together the vast number of medical, scientific, and literary sources into a manageable order.

Also, we profoundly appreciate the effort and expertise of Dorcas Demasio, the professional nutritionist who formulated the basic diets contained in this book.

Finally, we are grateful to Boston nutritionists, who reviewed all the diets and made some useful suggestions we have incorporated into the book.

Contents

The Brain Food Diet for Children

1

Are You Helping Your Child to Develop a Great Mind?

One day a few months ago, the mother of two young children, ages six months and two-and-a-half years, came into my office. As we were discussing her youngsters' health, I asked her—as I often do—what her goals were for her children.

Without any hesitation, she said, "I want each of them to have a great body and a great mind!"

Her response was typical. Almost every parent wants a healthy baby *and* a smart baby. But even though mothers and fathers want their sons and daughters to be highly intelligent, they have only a vague notion of how to go about achieving this result.

A few parents may get involved in extensive early education programs, such as those that teach very young children how to read, do math problems, speak additional languages, or otherwise get a head start on the subjects they may eventually learn in school. Other parents, taking a less formal but often even more effective approach, stress building a child's vocabulary by reading to him regularly and defining any difficult terms. They may also periodically drill him in his numbers and his letters.

Of course, many children seem to develop quickly into bright beings *without* any kind of special effort on the part of parents to enhance their intelligence. In those cases, friends and loved ones will say, more often than not, "Oh, Jimmy is smart, but he just takes after his folks. They've got an over-supply of brains!" Or, "Suzy is the spitting image of Aunt Maud, so you'd expect her to be sharp as a tack." In other words, they focus on the child's genes, on her possession of certain traits that bestow intelligence.

But what amazes me in all the concern about developing intelligent youngsters is the almost total neglect of what may be the most important factor of all—good nutrition. As a matter of fact, good nutrition in the first few years of life is probably the key building block for a person's later intelligence. If you feed your child the right foods in the first five years of life, you'll have laid an invaluable foundation for his ability to achieve and succeed in the future.

Indeed, the latest scientific research indicates that malnutrition—both of the mother during pregnancy and of the child during the first years of life—may jeopardize the brain's proper development. Two child nutrition experts, Dr. Myron Winick and Dr. Jo Anne Brasel of the Institute of Human Nutrition at Columbia University, have concluded that malnutrition early in life can:

• Retard brain growth;

- Reduce the rate of cell division in the brain;
- Slow the rate of formation of the protective sheath of the brain cells (or what is called the "myelin");
- Reduce the number of branches that grow out of each brain cell (the "dendritic arborizations"), which are thought to be key elements in the thinking process; and
- Change the process of the development of certain neural (nerve-related) hormones.

In some cases, these conditions may be reversible if the child embarks on a program of good nutrition. But in other instances they may not. For example, according to one recent report in *The New York Times* (April 7, 1983), a Harvard University health specialist, Dr. Larry Brown, testified thus before the Nutrition Subcommittee of the United States Senate: "A child's brain cannot wait for economic upswings."

Citing a study of 400 children five years of age and under at Boston City Hospital, Brown noted that doctors found three times the number of children they would have expected at the bottom of their growth charts. One report on the hearings observed that this age range is a "time when children are most susceptible to permanent brain damage from nutritional deprivation."

In a similar vein, Dr. Jean Mayer, the distinguished nutritionist and president of Tufts University, wrote in an article in *The Los Angeles Times* (April 7, 1983) that "we are being penny-wise and pound-foolish in our food stamp and other government nutritional programs." He went on to say that about 50 percent of the recipients of food stamps are children, and many others are pregnant women. As far as cost savings are concerned, he noted that the money it takes to feed children properly when they are very young is far less than the cost of treating them later for retardation and other forms of brain damage.

To be sure, the most serious impact of poor nutrition hits those in lower income brackets. But inadequate nutrition is not something that is limited to those with little money or poor education. In my own practice, I've found that even well-educated parents do not fully know their child's nutritional requirements. So, because most parents I've encountered at every income and educational level fail to feed their children the best possible "brain food diet," I decided that the time had come to write a practical book that would focus on the role of nutrition in a child's developing intelligence.

A fundamental principle in formulating this kind of program is that it must be a *child's* diet: That is, what the average child should eat will, most likely, not be at all appropriate for a healthy adult. In fact, the medical evidence shows that a young child's daily intake of food should in many ways be almost the *opposite* of that recommended for most adults.

For example, while adults are often told to reduce the amount of fats in their diets, the opposite is true for young children—especially those up to age three. Their growing brains need an abundance of fats, substances that nature has seen fit to provide in mother's milk, which is composed of more than 50 percent fat. By contrast, adults are often advised to limit their fat intake to no more than 30 percent of their daily calorie consumption.

In short, the special requirements of your child's growing brain demand that you should *not* feed your infant or toddler what the adults and older children in the family are eating. Instead, a separate approach to the very young child's diet is necessary. The model diets included in the later chapters of this book have been designed with these special needs in mind.

Furthermore, a young child's style of eating also has certain special characteristics. In particular, I have found that the three-meals-a-day tradition of most American families doesn't work for a young child whose stomach is relatively small and who consequently needs to eat more often than adults do. So, I would recommend that you think in terms of feeding your young boy or girl five meals a day instead of three. Again, the diets in this book have been constructed with this principle in mind.

But even as I offer this five-meal suggestion, I do so very cautiously. The reason is that flexibility is another vital principle in feeding the growing young brain. The most important thing for you to keep in mind is that *your child must get an adequate amount of food, no matter how you decide to go about it.* If six meals a day does the job better than five, then I'd say go for six. If four suits your child better, then make it four. If she typically needs to eat her final meal an hour before the rest of the family, then by all means do so.

Above all, don't substitute "junk food" or hollow calories for one of those important five meals. If you do, you'll most likely find your youngster's mental acumen taking a nosedive.

For example, one mother recently came into my office with her little daughter, Mary, who was just a few months short of three. The main problem was that the girl had been acting increasingly agitated, quarrelsome, and fretful. Also, she was completely unwilling to sit still long enough for her mother to read to her. As a result, she had almost no knowledge of the nursery rhymes, fairy tales, and Bible stories—and the accompanying vocabulary—which her peers were beginning to master. The mother worried that Mary might be hyperactive, mental disturbed, or otherwise emotionally unhealthy.

I did a number of tests but couldn't find anything, so the mother and I sat down and I began to question her about some of the customs around the home—especially the family eating habits. During this conversation, I learned what I had suspected all along: The child was hungry.

You see, often, when Mary became fretful between meals, her mother gave her soft drinks, corn chips, candy, cookies, or some other hollow-calorie snack. Then, later, the mother would serve an attractive meal, but Mary would just pick at it. The youngster never ate adequately at the family's traditional mealtime because of the junk foods she filled her stomach with during the odd hours when she was hungry.

My "prescription" was fairly clear-cut in this case. I told the mother to toss out the junk food, and plan five meals a day for Mary, with the meals spaced about three hours apart. And I put the little girl on the kind of brain food diet that has been included in this book.

The result? The girl's disposition improved; she soon developed a relatively calm, easy-going manner; and she was able to sit still for twenty to thirty minutes at a time as her mother read to her.

So, in Mary's case, the right food plan made her more open and receptive to intellectual activities and interests. In addition, it is likely that the general physical development of her brain got back on the right track. You see, the most significant brain growth in human beings takes place up to about age five. This means that it's essential for the right kinds of foods, those that are going to promote brain growth, to get into a child's system as early as possible.

At this stage of medical research, it is not completely clear what the precise impact may be of mild or marginally adequate nutrition. But nutrition for the brain, like nutrition for other parts of the body, most probably functions on a kind of scale: In other words, if your child gets only adequate nutrition, it is likely that the structures in his brain will not develop as well as they might otherwise with the best possible food program.

There have been no definitive long-term (or "longitudinal") studies on this subject, and it is likely there may never be. The reason is that there are several deep-rooted problems with testing different nutrition programs on youngsters at such a young age. One set of difficulties is ethical: It would be morally questionable to set aside one "control" group of youngsters who must remain malnourished and then provide another group, with whom they are to be compared, with superior nutrition. The dilemma is, of course: How do you choose which children get good nutrition and which don't? That is a problem that our society is not inclined to explore.

But there are also problems on the purely practical level. Currently, we just don't have any tests that can do a good job of evaluating the intelligence of children who are two, three, or even four years of age in relation to future performance. Brain power develops at different rates in different children. So, a child who tests low on the scale at age three may be above average at age four, just because of the genetic programming in his body that causes his brain to expand at a certain speed.

Or you may have a very bright child at age three who is emotionally immature. He may be quite capable of answering any question on a standardized test, but he may not be able to sit still long enough to finish it. I'm reminded of one little girl who went in to be tested for a preschool program for gifted children. She knew the answers to most of the questions, but halfway through the test she began to get silly. She pointed to the answers with her nose and ears, and the man conducting the test apparently didn't understand what was happening. As a result, he gave her a low mark when she should have been right at the top.

So it's difficult, if not impossible, to measure the precise impact of various influences—including nutrition—on a child's intelligence at a very young age. But despite the lack of exact measurements, the weight of medical evidence does seem to indicate that a child's diet *will* make a big difference in the development of his brain power. So it's very important that you, as a parent, pay particular attention to three stages in your child's development up to about age five. These are:

- **Pregnancy:** In our weight-conscious society, mothers need to understand that the state of their nutrition will affect their child's brain. The brain of the unborn child needs certain nutrients to develop properly, and so the mother-to-be should plan her diet carefully during pregnancy. In fact, it's also important for the woman to plan her diet *before* pregnancy. If you've been dieting and weigh less than what the latest weight charts or your doctor say you should weigh, then it's important to start eating properly and reach your ideal weight before you conceive.

- **From birth to age three:** This is the most important period for a child's brain growth. A "growth spurt" occurs during these three years that brings your youngster's brain up to about 80 percent of its adult size. Breast milk has traditionally been the best brain food during this stage of life. As we'll see later, in many societies at an earlier period of history, it was normal for mothers to breast-feed their children up to about age three.

Although such a long period at the breast isn't usually feasible these days, I certainly recommend breast-feeding for at least the first six months of life. So the diet I've devised, while it is well balanced in all respects to promote a child's growth, has been formulated to come as close as possible to the constituency of mother's milk. This means, as I've already indicated, that your child at this time of life should be eating a diet that's relatively high in fats and lower than typical adult diets in carbohydrates and protein.

- **From age three to five:** Most of the rest of your child's brain development, including the important sheathing of brain cells that may be a key component in physical coordination, takes place during this final period. As a result, I recommend that children up to age five stay on a diet similar to that of the first three years, with appropriate adjustments for increased calories as the youngster gets bigger.

  And one other thing: During this preschool stage of life, children often become as influenced by television advertising as do adults. So it's important for you, the parent, to take a firm hand in limiting or eliminating junk food and in keeping your child on the straight-and-narrow path of a solid brain food diet.

  As I did with the little girl, Mary, I would suggest that you think in terms of about five meals a day for your child. At least two of those meals should be scheduled for your youngster's typical snack time. A glass of whole milk or some other nutritious brain food at these between-meal points will do much more for the development of those young brain cells than a sack of potato chips!

From the years that I've spent counseling concerned parents and treating children's health problems, I know the development of a youngster's intelligence is an extremely important and sensitive matter. Every mother or father wants his children to be as bright as possible because a superior intellect is often associated with greater opportunities and satisfaction in life. The material that I am presenting to you in this book is both hard facts and specific programs to help you increase the odds that your child's brain will develop *physically* to its maximum potential. After that, it will be up to you to provide the home environment and educational opportunities to transform that physical base—those brain cells with their various electrical and chemical connections—into the most effective tools for success in life.

In the ensuing chapters, I'll explain in more detail precisely what is going on in your child's brain at different stages of his life. Lastly, you'll be provided with a comprehsive set of diets for youngsters at every age level, from their time in the womb through age five.

But first, it's important to examine some myths and "old wives' tales" about intelligence, some of which have been floating around for centuries. What we are concerned with in this book is medical facts, and I want to be sure you can separate those facts from invalid beliefs or highly questionable folklore.

2

Fact and Folklore About Brain Power

Throughout the ages, mankind has been preoccupied with intelligence, and especially with the influence, financial and otherwise, that a person with an exceptional brain can command.

You may recall that King Solomon asked God first for wisdom—or, as the Bible says, "a discerning heart to govern your people and to distinguish between right and wrong." God was pleased, and replied, "I will give you a wise and discerning heart, so that there will never have been anyone like you, nor will there ever be. Moreover, I will give you what you have not asked for—both riches and honor—so that in your lifetime you will have no equal among kings." (1 Kings 3:9–13, New International Version).

Ever since that point, a premium has been placed on brain power. Of course, superior "mental horsepower" has always been the quality that makes human beings distinctive and dominant among living creatures. Moreover, the human being who has high intelligence—along with the will and ability to use it—often rises to a position of leadership and superior achievement. It is no wonder that philosophers, scientists, and educators, as well as astute parents, have long been enthralled by the question of what makes some people smarter than others.

Because of the importance of the human mind, a wealth of opinion has arisen on the subject of intelligence. Just ask anyone on the street what makes a person intelligent, and he or she will probably give you a quick answer—whether it's a paraphrase of a current pop psychologist's theory or a reflection of a bit of folk wisdom that great-grandma used to impart.

Concern about how to improve the individual's level of mental ability—or "brain power," if you will—has intensified in recent decades with the increasing stress on specialized technological and professional skills. Everyone has a pet theory about what he or she can do, or should have done, to improve skills and intellectual capacities, and hence his or her position in life. But there's nothing new about this impulse toward identifying some kind of magic formula for a mighty mind. In fact, outrageous and not-so-outrageous beliefs about the sources of high intelligence have been around for centuries.

One of the myths that intrigues me personally, perhaps because of my interest in nutrition, is the idea that in order to *develop* brains, you should *eat* brains. Of course, that doesn't necessarily mean human brains, though in some primitive, cannibalistic societies, human brains were considered a delicacy! Some prehistorians have even suggested that primitive Neanderthal man was cannibalistic, and that his intelligence increased and his evolutionary status advanced as he consumed the brains of other Neanderthals!

As bizarre as this concept may seem, there may even be a little bit of truth in it. For example, studies of tiny organisms called planaria have shown that when one of these creatures eats another that has been conditioned to perform certain movements, the first "cannibalistic" planarian often acquires the same abilities as the second, conditioned creature.

Of course, this is not the same thing as having one creature eat the brains of another because simple creatures like planaria cannot be said to have brains in the same sense that higher animals do. But scientific studies show there is real basis for eating a food that is a good source of nutrients for a part of the body you are trying to strengthen or improve.

Some other rather strange ideas have emerged in the past as to how people can enhance their mental capacities. The rather bizarre suggestion that brain power can be improved by eating the brains of another animal, including another human being, is only the tip of the folk-belief iceberg. Consider the merits of some other notions that in many cases are equally unusual.

- **The color of a wet nurse's hair affects a child's brain power:** In the nineteenth century when it was fashionable for women *not* to nurse their babies, young mothers hired wet nurses to do the job for them. Naturally, there was a great "to do" over the selection of a wet nurse. And the idea was generally accepted that brunettes made better wet nurses than blondes and redheads.

  Could there possibly be any reason for such a prejudice? Yes, indeed! Many people in those days were convinced that hair color reflected a person's temperament. Brunettes were thought to have the most stable personalities, the strongest physical and emotional make-up, and, consequently, the healthiest milk.

The common wisdom was that redheads should be avoided as wet nurses because, as one nineteenth-century American writer named Dewees put it:

> There may be certain moral qualities that may unfit them for the office of nurses; they are certainly of sanguine temperament, and this temperament has attached to it great irritability of temper as one of its characteristics—hence, in a moral point of view, their unfitness as protectors of young children.

Similarly, blondes were thought to have a more passionate character than brunettes. As a consequence, people tended to think their milk could deteriorate under mental excitement. Charles H. F. Routh, a prolific nineteenth-century English nutrition writer, said that in extreme cases "the milk of blondes has been known to produce the death of the infants."

Brunettes, in contrast, were supposed to have a more "melancholic" temperament, which was regarded as just the thing infants needed to develop properly. As Routh wrote:

> Their milk is richer, and a precocious child is, as it were, restrained by this milk from over excitement in its mental manifestations. Its body has time to be formed and to develop itself before it is exhausted by undue psychical excitement, and a stronger child is the result.

While wrong-headed in most respects, there was a seed of truth in these nineteenth-century ideas. As we'll see shortly, the richness of the mother's milk *is* important to brain development. The problem with the folk wisdom is that this richness apparently has nothing to do with the color of the mother's or the wet nurse's hair!

- **Feeding children fish will make them smart:** This conviction comes from the notion that fish is "brain food." And it's true that in a certain sense and in certain cases, it is. In the days before iodized salt, many land-locked people suffered from iodine deficiency—a lack that causes the thyroid gland to enlarge, the production of the thyroid hormone to decrease, and mental functioning to slow down.

  When iodine-deficient people eat fish—and specifically salt-water fish—this process can be reversed. They begin to feel better generally and become more alert. The reason for this dramatic change is simple: Salt-water fish are a good source of iodine and can therefore cure iodine deficiency and restore normal mental functioning.

  So, in this sense, at least, fish can act as a brain food. But don't expect your children to be brilliant just because you feed them a steady diet of tuna salad. It takes a more comprehensive approach to a child's diet at the right age to achieve any sort of permanent impact on brain power.

- **Eggs are an important "brain food":** People in various cultures have come up with the idea that eating eggs will make a child "smart." Modern medical research indicates there may be a great deal of truth to this notion. Eggs are one of the brain foods I recommend for preschool children, especially because of the fat contained in them.

Also, as Carol Ann Rinzler notes in *The Dictionary Of Medical Folklore*, eggs, meat, and fish "may help stimulate the brain or at least transmit its messages to the body." She argues that these foods are rich in a fatty substance called lecithin, a source of choline, which, in turn, produces acetylcholine.

"Acetylcholine is one of many chemicals which act as transmitters for brain impulses within the body," Rinzler says. "Scientists have speculated that insufficient quantities of acetylcholine in the body may be responsible for mental problems, such as manic behavior, and for loss of memory."

• **A child will be more intelligent if his mother engages in cultural activities during pregnancy:** There is some evidence that babies can hear sounds in the womb. For example, a number of pregnant women have reported that they detect certain types of movement by the fetus in response to music that is playing nearby. If this is the case, who is to say that music cannot in some way affect a baby's ability in later life to respond to or even appreciate music? At this point, we just don't know.

When it comes to museums, however, it's probably wise not to expect too much! Such cultural activities as a trip to an exhibit of painting or sculpture can certainly stimulate your intelligence. But any beneficial impact on your unborn child will most likely have to wait until he's been out of the womb for a few years.

• **Talking to your baby in the womb will increase**

her vocabulary: There's certainly no hard evidence for the validity of this belief. But I do know some parents who have tried talking to the fetus through the wall of the womb, and they claim their children are more verbal than average and more responsive to reason and the spoken word at a relatively young age.

I seriously doubt, however, that there is any chance you'll increase your child's vocabulary by this practice.

- **Painting the nursery yellow will spur your child's intelligence:** For centuries people have said that color can have a powerful effect on human behavior. And there may just be something to this notion.

According to some recent studies conducted at the San Bernardino County Probation Department in California, manic and psychotic juveniles tend to relax and fall asleep—sometimes within ten minutes—when they are put into a cell that is painted "bubblegum" pink. It's been argued too that the colors orange and red act as appetite stimulants and as gregarious influences that tend to draw people together. Perhaps the orange motif has had something to do with the success of those Howard Johnson's restaurants!

So what about yellow? Can this hue enhance intelligence?

Popular writers who focus on the effects of environment on behavior and learning ability contend that yellow does indeed awaken one's mental faculties and help conquer negativity and nervousness. But whether or not this color should be used in the nursery is another matter. In fact, some authorities feel yellow may be too exciting for a child's bedroom, even though it may be just right in the study or in any other place where you want to cultivate an upbeat, alert, creative attitude.

The impact of the type of lighting people use in their homes has also been a source of much speculation and theorizing. Some writers have even suggested, for example, that ultraviolet light can spur a child's IQ. But like ideas about color, the full implication of this idea remains to be proven.

These, then, are a few of the traditions and beliefs that have attempted to explain why some children turn out to be smarter than others. But they are only a small part of the network of fact and fantasy that has evolved over the years on the subject. For example, just as there has been all sorts of speculation about the causes of intelligence, there have also been many "tests" that have emerged to evaluate how smart a child is becoming—or how well the assumed "causes" of intelligence are working.

Here are a few "intelligence tests" that will give you an idea of how the fancies of men and women, both in the past and the present, have taken flight on this subject.

Test Number One:
A Child Who Has Fast Hand Reactions
Also Tends to Have a Quick Mind

During the nineteenth century, scholars exploring the emerging discipline of psychology began to search for ways to determine the intelligence of young children and students. They assumed in many cases that there had to be a correlation between the child's physical reactions and his ability to think quickly and effectively.

As a result, they tried such tests as measuring the

speed of a tapped pencil, the quickness of hand movements in response to outside stimulation, and the overall sensitivity to touch. But these lines of inquiry resulted in a dead end because there was no difference in classroom performance between those students whose physical reactions were slow and those whose reactions were fast.

Test Number Two:
Children Who Walk and Talk
Early Are Smarter Than Others

Although precocious walking and talking have traditionally been matters of pride for parents, these activities do not necessarily indicate superior intelligence. When parents who come in to see me reveal they are worried because their son or daughter isn't walking or talking as early as the neighborhood children, I ask them first what the rest of their family was like at that age. When did their child's siblings and cousins start walking and talking? How about the parents and grandparents, if anyone can remember that far back?

You see, many times, the tendency to walk or talk early on is a genetic characteristic, a family trait involving the nervous system, which develops or matures at a certain preprogrammed point and which has nothing to do with overall intelligence. In most cases, walking and talking is a matter of this kind of development and not a clear-cut indicator of brain power.

Test Number Three:
A High Aptitude Test Score in the
Preschool Years Means Success
and Achievement Throughout Life

These days, even nursery schools and other preschool educational centers interviewing youngsters who are two and three years old may give various tests that are supposed to show something about the child's ability to perform in a classroom situation. These tests may be as informal as having the child try to put together simple puzzles or asking her to distinguish between objects scattered on a table. Or they may be as formal as the series of "Circus" tests put out for preschoolers by the Educational Testing Service, where the child is asked to demonstrate his ability to distinguish between characteristics on cartoonlike panels containing line drawings of people and objects.

Certainly, some of these evaluations—especially those that have been devised by the best-equipped testing institutions—show something about the child's potential to perform in a certain educational environment at a particular point in the youngster's process of development. But it may be impossible to predict accurately from such tests how a young child will do in later life.

In fact, even at later ages, intelligence examinations like IQ tests are inadequate for predicting achievement during the adult years. For example, according to research done by Dr. Robert B. McCall at the Fels Research Institute in Yellow Springs, Ohio, there is a 60 percent chance at age seven of predicting performance in adult life from a child's IQ; an 80 percent chance at age thirteen; and a 60 percent chance at age eighteen.

So, a high IQ doesn't necessarily mean your child will do well later. And an average or low IQ doesn't consign any youngster to failure.

It is also important to realize that an IQ or other intelligence test score can change over the years. Family life, education, and nutrition can raise or lower a child's IQ by at least 10 points and sometimes by 20.

Test Number Four:
Bright Children Have Larger
Heads and Higher Foreheads

During at least the last couple of centuries, educators have tried to show that the larger the head and the brain, the smarter the individual. While none of these tests have ever been proven conclusive, there is some evidence in favor of brain size (though not high foreheads) as a measure of intelligence.

When R. E. Passingham of Oxford University measured the cranial capacity of people with known IQs, he found a slight connection between skull size and intelligence. Or, as Passingham wrote, when the height of the individuals was taken into account, "it was possible to demonstrate a statistically significant, but very slight, relation between brain size and occupational group."

So, as odd as it may seem, there may be something to the idea that large heads and big brains mean greater personal ability. As a matter of fact, pediatricians keep close track of the development of head size as one of the measurements of normal growth in a child. And as we watch the head expand, one of the considerations on many of our minds is that the intellectual capacity of the youngster is expanding as well.

At this point, you may be wondering if there is any valid way to determine your own child's head and brain development at an early age. The most precise way to check on this is to ask your pediatrician how your child's head development is doing in relation to other children his age.

The doctor should be measuring your child's head regularly, and he should also be using a chart showing how your child's head compares with other children on a percentile basis. In other words, if your youngster is above the 50th percentile, that means that his head is larger than half the other children his age. And if he's below the 50th percentile, his head is in the smaller half.

But remember: A key consideration is the overall size of your child, not the comparative size of his head. If he tends to be small for his age, then he is naturally probably going to have a smaller head. In fact, he may be in the 40th percentile for head circumference and still be a genius just because he tends to be a small person.

In addition to questioning your doctor, there are a few practical tests you can conduct on your own.

For example, it is helpful to informally monitor the circumference of your child's head in relation to his or her body size. Because the soft spot doesn't close and the skull is very thin until the child is eighteen months to two years of age, any measurement of the head at this stage is predominantly a measurement of brain size. If the size is excessively large or small in proportion to the body, that can often be a sign of brain abnormality.

There are two easy ways to do a crude but reasonably effective check by yourself:

- **Notice the ease with which T-shirts and other pullovers slip on and off your child's head:** Clothing manufacturers establish the size of pullovers according to the 50th percentile of a particular age group. So, if you have great difficulty in getting shirts on and off your youngster—or if they go over his head quite easily—you might ask your physician to check him out more closely. The probable reason for any difficulty or ease with clothing is the fact that your child is generally large or small for his age, and his unusual head size most likely has nothing to do with brain power.

- **Measure your child's head with a tape measure:**

Just wrap the tape around the middle of his forehead and across the little knot on the back of the head. Then compare this figure and your child's overall length with the charts included on pages 00 through 00.

If there is a wide variation between the percentiles of body size and brain size, you should discuss this fact with your physician. In other words, if your measurements show the 75th percentile for the child's body and the 25th percentile for the brain, that would be cause for a professional pediatric evaluation. Remember, though, that slight variations between brain size and body length in the percentile readings are normal.

So, if your boy or girl has a slightly larger brain size in proportion to body size, he or she may turn out to be fairly intelligent. But what we're talking about here is *raw* intelligence: In other words, your child may have the basic mental equipment to be a high achiever. But without the motivation, self-confidence, inner drive, and all the other psychological factors that don't depend on intelligence, that bright mind may not take him or her very far.

Test Number Five:
You Can Tell How Intelligent a
Child Is by Watching the Eyes

At first glance, this may appear a far too subjective "test" to take seriously. But actually, watching a child's responses to the world around her can be one of the best indicators of mental acuity.

A child's eyes, more than those of many adults, may show unveiled anxiety, fear, joy, and curiosity. I always watch to see if a infant notices an object I'm holding in

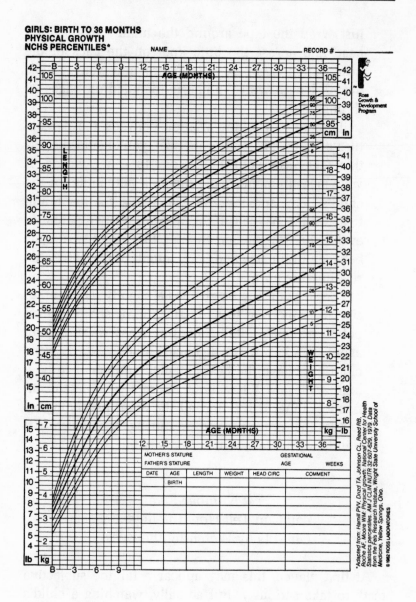

GIRLS: BIRTH TO 36 MONTHS
PHYSICAL GROWTH
NCHS PERCENTILES*

GIRLS: BIRTH TO 36 MONTHS
PHYSICAL GROWTH
NCHS PERCENTILES*

NAME_____ RECORD #_____

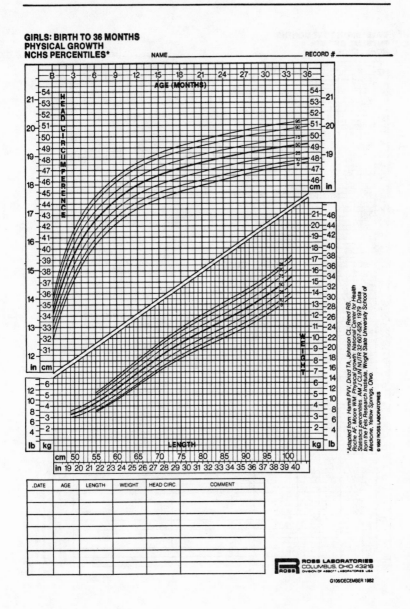

.DATE	AGE	LENGTH	WEIGHT	HEAD CIRC	COMMENT

*Adapted from Hamill PVV, Drizd TA, Johnson CL, Reed RB, Roche AF, Moore WM. Physical growth: National Center for Health Statistics percentiles. AM J CLIN NUTR 32:607-629, 1979. Data from the Fels Research Institute, Wright State University School of Medicine, Yellow Springs, Ohio.

© 1982 ROSS LABORATORIES

ROSS LABORATORIES
COLUMBUS, OHIO 43216
DIVISION OF ABBOTT LABORATORIES USA

G106/DECEMBER 1982

BOYS: BIRTH TO 36 MONTHS
PHYSICAL GROWTH
NCHS PERCENTILES*

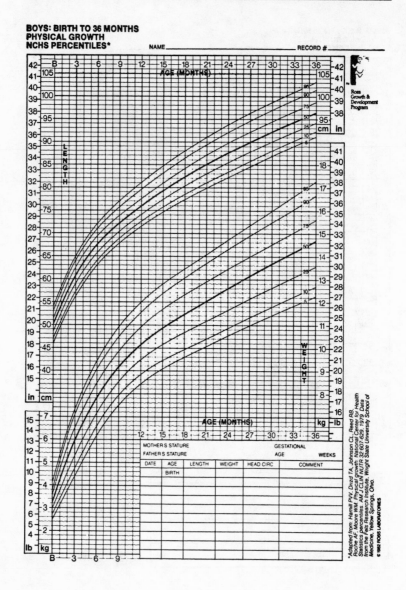

BOYS: BIRTH TO 36 MONTHS
PHYSICAL GROWTH
NCHS PERCENTILES*   NAME_____ RECORD #_____

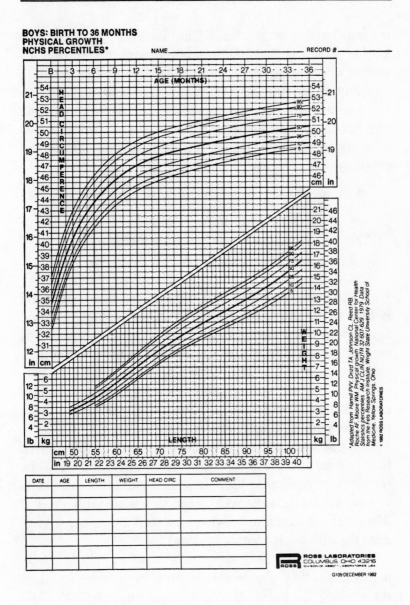

*Adapted from Hamill PVV, Drizd TA, Johnson CL, Reed RB, Roche AF, Moore WM. Physical growth National Center for Health Statistics percentiles AM J CLIN NUTR 32:607-629 1979. Data from the Fels Research Institute, Wright State University School of Medicine, Yellow Springs, Ohio
© 1982 ROSS LABORATORIES*

DATE	AGE	LENGTH	WEIGHT	HEAD CIRC	COMMENT

ROSS LABORATORIES
COLUMBUS, OHIO 43216
DIVISION OF ABBOTT LABORATORIES, USA

G105/DECEMBER 1982

my hand and tries to grab it. That indicates an aggressive kind of curiosity that I believe bodes well for future intellectual accomplishments. I also watch a child's reaction to shiny or moving objects in various parts of the room. An intent, curious gaze, especially in an infant of six months to a year, demonstrates natural alertness and tells me that the young brain is probably developing properly.

Test Number Six:
Attention Span is a Barometer of
Brain Power

Many authorities feel that a good test of a good mind is the child's attention span. To a great extent, I would agree with this idea. For example, most two-year-olds can sit down and engage themselves with another person, a toy, or some other center of interest for a reasonable period of time. It is quite likely that more intelligent children can concentrate on such tasks longer than those with less natural mental ability.

To test your own child's development in this regard in an informal way, ask yourself: How long can she remain at a particular task? Is it a constructive task, or is it meaningless? How well does she play with others? Also, can she imitate what adults and other older children do with a fair amount of ease?

Of course, not all these questions relate only to intelligence. But they do relate to how well your child is responding to stimulation from his environment. And between one and three years of age, his response to such stimulation may be one of the best indicators of intelligence that is available.

Up to this point, we've been talking about tradition and popular belief almost as much as about the solid scientific basis for helping your child to maximize his brain power. It is true that there is still room for speculation and even for folk wisdom because much is, even now, unknown about the development of the brain in those crucial early years, when the foundations of intelligence are laid.

But despite our limitations, scientific evidence has been pointing more and more in recent years toward nutrition as the key element in the early development of a person's intelligence. Now, let us take a closer look at how the right kind of food can produce that miracle—your child's mind.

3

The Miracle
of Your Child's
Young Mind

Take a few moments to study your young son or
daughter. What do you see that you like? Perhaps it's her bright winsome smile. Or maybe it's his
smooth faultless skin. Or it could be that full head of
curly black hair.

There is certainly reason for you to be proud of your
youngster's physical looks and friendly personality.
Those qualities will stand him in good stead in years to
come. But an even more important factor in determining
the shape of his future—a factor that most parents I know
don't seriously consider until it's too late—is what's
going on inside that little head. In fact, parents, even
those who have a high level of education and should
know better, are often woefully ignorant and neglectful
about their child's brain development. They'll comb his
hair or dress her up in an adorable frock. But the atten-

tion they pay to the child's intelligence is haphazard at best.

As I've already indicated, the early years of a child's life, from the womb until about age five, are the most decisive in the physical development of the brain. Yet here is the sort of thing that I encounter daily in my pediatric practice:

- One expectant mother was obsessed with staying slim even as her stomach began to show in the fifth month of pregnancy. She had a number of complications in her pregnancy, primarily as a result of her failure to eat properly and maintain sufficient weight. As a result, she had to be hospitalized several times before childbirth. When her baby was born, he weighed only four and a half pounds—the low weight being apparently a direct result of the mother's poor nutrition during pregnancy. The youngster was rather sickly and grew slowly, and I feared that with his comparatively small head size, he may have experienced some stunting of brain growth.

  When the woman and child came under my care, I immediately recommended breast-feeding and put the woman on a solid nursing (or lactation) diet, with nutritional supplements. The child began to grow faster over a period of a few months, and I noticed some improvement in his alertness. But the "jury is still out" as far as the final impact on this child's intelligence is concerned.

  Although poor nutrition during pregnancy means danger to the development of a child's brain, any damage done to the brain cells can often be reversed by good nutrition just after birth. But my feeling is, why take chances? One-sixth of your

child's brain development will take place in the
womb; all of his brain cells will be formed there;
and permanent damage is possible after the sixth or
seventh month of pregnancy. So why not stack the
odds in your child's favor? Treat her as though she
really is your child while she is still kicking inside
you, and feed her brain with the right diet by eating
properly yourself.

• Another mother with a cute two-year-old came into
my office and asked, "Should I place Millicent on
skim milk or low-fat milk? I was reading the other
day that children can develop problems with fat,
even at a very young age—so should I keep her away
from whole milk?"

I told her in no uncertain terms, *"No!"* I know
that some physicians recommend low-fat milk for a
child, even at the toddler stage. But I believe the
clear message from current medical knowledge is
that the brains of very young children need fats
which are present in whole milk.

I knew what this young mother was thinking:
Everyone in her family was quite athletic and concerned about their health and looks. Millicent
tended to be a little heavy because she was large-
boned; and so I suspected the mother was project-
ing her own consciousness about her weight and
physical fitness onto her daughter. The problem
was that the adult diet and conditioning program
that other members of the family pursued would not
be appropriate for such a young child.

• But there's a flip side to this milk issue: Another
patient of mine, a two-year-old named Sarah, was
quite lethargic—certainly not at all the energetic,
vibrant person you'd expect someone her age to be.

She had a sweet disposition and was rather plump, but she was also too pale.

After a physical examination, I asked her mother about the child's diet and learned that she was getting *too much* whole milk. That is, she wasn't getting enough fruits, vegetables, meats and other foods that would provide her with the iron that she needed to keep her energy up. In short, she was anemic because of a mild iron deficiency.

When we adjusted Sarah's diet, she soon perked up and became what I can only describe as "sparky." Her activity level and curiosity about her surroundings increased perceptibly, and she began to learn more quickly and interact with people much more readily.

- The same sort of correlation between good nutrition and mental alertness applies to older children: As a consultant for a preschool program for underprivileged children, I found that a number had a variety of personality and emotional problems that made it impossible for them to learn anything in a classroom environment. Many of these youngsters, who were three to four years old, were very aggressive, agitated, or argumentative on the one hand; or were totally "zonked out," sluggish, or whiny on the other.

  After conducting a survey of their family backgrounds, including their eating habits, I discovered that many of the children regularly ate little or nothing for breakfast. So we arranged to give them a full breakfast immediately after they arrived at the program—including eggs, fruit, cheese, whole milk, french toast, and other dishes which I have identified over the years as "brain food."

  Within days after we had made this adjustment

in their diets, we noticed a clear difference in the youngsters' behavior and attentiveness in class. The agitated children calmed down and lost much of their sense of confusion. They were also able to comprehend the subjects in their nursery school class and take on social relationships in a more organized way. The excessively lethargic children, on the other hand, perked up, began to contribute more at "story time," showed a greater interest in working puzzles, and generally became more involved in the activities around them.

• An older child, about five years old, was a "holy terror" the first time he came into my office. He couldn't sit still for more than ten seconds, was quarrelsome, and was completely unable to concentrate on any conversation that I would try to strike up with him. His mother indicated that his behavior was sometimes so bizarre he almost seemed to be on drugs. He would slide and chase around the room at a breakneck clip, as though he were possessed. He was also completely unable to concentrate on his kindergarten studies, and his parents were quite worried about his ability to function effectively when he entered the first grade the following year.

In questioning the mother about his diet, I learned that instead of eating a nutritious brain food snack as one of his five meals a day, he was filling up on chocolate and various soft drinks. I suspected that his main problem was the caffeine in these substances, and so I told the mother, "Let's try an experiment. Don't give him any chocolate or soft drinks for the next two weeks and see how he reacts. Give me a call after the two-week period is up."

Sure enough, he calmed down almost immediately. He also became a much better student and made the transition to the first grade much more smoothly.

When you consider examples like these, one important question often comes to mind: How much of the damage to a child's mind due to poor nutrition is temporary, and how much is permanent?

Certainly, there is at least a temporary impact on mental functioning in many of these cases because you can see an immediate improvement in the ability to learn and communicate after the child goes on a proper brain food diet. But there is also evidence that inadequate nutrition, especially over a relatively long period of time, will cause permanent impairment of a child's mental abilities.

For example, consider some studies done on Korean orphans who came to the United States several years ago at a young age. One group of the orphans suffered from malnourishment during the first year of life. A second group of Korean orphans had been moderately nourished; and a third group was well-nourished. All groups were adopted before age three by American families and were put on relatively equal, nutritionally healthy diets.

The malnourished group was tested later and was found to have IQ and achievement test scores somewhat lower than average for children in the United States. The other two groups—those who had originally been moderately nourished and well-nourished—scored even higher than the American norms.

Some experts say studies of the Korean orphans show that malnutrition may be reversible, since the malnourished youngsters scored at least close to the normal level

for children in a broad population that had been generally well-nourished. But others have suggested that since
all these children came from the same cultural environment, the relatively superior performance of the youngsters who had always been well-nourished shows that
malnutrition at a early age may do irreparable damage.

Or, as Dr. Merrill Read, chief of the Growth and
Development Branch of the National Institute of Child
Health and Human Development, puts it: "These observations [of Korean orphans] suggest that malnourished
children, even though they are not retarded in later life,
are never able to achieve their full intellectual potential."

One weakness in these studies is that the children
couldn't be tested before they came to the States to see
how much their scores had gone up after they arrived
here. Indeed, as I've already indicated, there are no completely reliable intelligence tests for children who are
barely in the toddler stage of life. So, it's not absolutely
definite what effect malnutrition had on the Korean
orphans. But even with the lack of perfect controls and
the impossibility of determining the precise degree to
which the children's brain power improved with good
nutrition, this study does suggest that it's quite likely that
good nutrition helps in enhancing intelligence—and in
preventing permanent mental impairment.

Another study focused on groups of undernourished
children who were over two years old. The researchers
found that improving the diet increased the average IQ
by 18 points. Also, the earlier the nutritional therapy was
given, the greater was the rise in IQ. After age four, however, the rise in IQ was insignificant.

Such results certainly suggest that the adverse effects
of malnutrition are reversible—but only up to a certain
age, probably four or five. Once the child reaches that
ceiling age, the effects of prior malnutrition may become
permanent.

At this point, an objection may be raised that I have mentioned briefly before, but that warrants further discussion: That is, most of these studies have focused on children who were truly malnourished—not on those who were from middle-class families who may have been getting diets that were a little out of balance. So, some may suggest that cases of severe malnutrition can't be compared with the average diet of the average family in an affluent Western society.

My own feeling, though, is that it's likely there are *degrees* of damage from improper nutrition, even among those who might be considered well-fed in our society. For example, assume that two families may have the money and the social and educational background to give their children equal intellectual advantages. One family pays close attention to providing an excellent diet for their preschool children—a diet that stresses those foods that have the best chance of enhancing brain power. The other family, in contrast, does little to promote good nutrition and provides only a fair diet.

In such a case, the preschool children from the nutrition-conscious family should have at least a slight intellectual edge on those from the second: That is, the first group of youngsters should come closer to realizing their maximum intelligence potential because the developing branches, sheaths, and cells in their brains have been provided with better nourishment.

Now, in more specific terms, let's take a look at what takes place in your youngster's head at different stages of his brain development. It is from the later months of pregnancy through about age five that your child's most significant brain growth takes place. It is also during that period that permanent damage to one degree or another is most likely to occur as a result of poor nutrition.

To understand this process better, let's trace the actual development of the brain of your child—whom we'll call "Jimmy"—from the moment of conception up to about age five. Of course, "Jimmy" could as easily be "Jane." There's no difference in the way the brain of a little boy or girl grows. So, if you have a daughter, feel free to substitute "Jane" for "Jimmy" in the following narrative.

In the first few weeks after conception, little Jimmy doesn't really have a brain at all—just a mass of undifferentiated cells. But by the time he reaches his full size as a young adult, he'll be the proud possessor of a brain that is perhaps the most amazing, intricate organ in all creation.

Jimmy's adult human brain will be composed mainly of DNA (or deoxyribonucleic acid, which is the basic molecular component of heredity in living organisms); RNA (ribonucleic acid, the complex, single-stranded molecule that aids the synthesis of DNA and protein in living organisms); and various proteins, many of which are high in fat content. His fully-grown brain may range in size up to 2,000 cubic centimeters.

To reach this size, Jimmy's brain goes through three main stages of growth: (1) *brain cell formation*, when those general, undefined cells that appear after conception become brain cells; (2) *brain cell division*, when one of Jimmy's brain cells divides into two, those two into four, and so on; and (3) *brain cell development*, which takes place from the last three months of your pregnancy up until Jimmy reaches about age five. During this third stage, Jimmy's brain cells stop dividing and complex chemical and structural changes in his brain start to occur. This final stage also includes an all-important "growth spurt" phase, which usually takes place from about the seventh month of pregnancy to the third year of life.

Now here, in more intimate detail, is what happens

during each of these three stages of Jimmy's brain growth.

Jimmy's Brain During the First Three Months in Your Womb: Cell Formation

The process of brain cell formation, which is the first stage of any child's brain growth, starts at conception and ends in the third month of pregnancy. What you eat during this period determines what your growing unborn son eats as a tiny fetus.

Jimmy's nervous system (his brain, spinal cord, and nerves) begins as a flat sheet of general cells called the *neural plate*. As food comes in and development proceeds, this plate starts to fold over and form what is called the *neural groove*. Finally, it closes entirely to become the *neural tube*. From this tube, the spinal cord and all three brain lobes (the midbrain, hindbrain, and forebrain) emerge—like a kind of tree topped by boughs and branches.

During his first three months in the womb, Jimmy's brain undergoes what scientists call *cellular differentiation*. This means that throughout your unborn child's little body, general cells become specialized brain cells, eye cells, skin cells, and so on. In other words, the general cells "differentiate" into cells with a more specific purpose.

One important feature of this first stage of Jimmy's brain development is that there is a definite time limit during which it takes place. If brain cells are removed or damaged during the differentiation period—say, in the neural plate which eventually serves as the basis for forming the eye and forebrain—neighboring cells will quickly "step in" and replace the missing or damaged area. But if cells are removed from the same area at a *later* date, when all the cells in Jimmy's body have already differentiated, a defect will appear in either his eye or forebrain.

So, to get your child off to a good start in life, it is certainly important for you to eat well from the very beginning of your pregnancy. But there does seem to be less likelihood of permanent damage to your child from poor nutrition in the first stage of his development—and especially when the differentiation of his brain cells is just beginning. The greatest danger arises after the differentiation of brain cells has been completed.

Jimmy's Brain in the Second Stage of Your Pregnancy: Cell Division

Every healthy brain is made up of millions of brain cells, which are actually nerve cells called *neurons*. The neuron has three main parts: (1) the *axon* (an extension of a neuron that resembles an extension cord leading away from an electrical outlet); (2) the *cell body*; and (3) the *axon terminal*.

It is during this second stage of brain growth, in the second trimester of your pregnancy, that most of Jimmy's neurons are created through rapid cell division. That is, one cell quickly divides into two; those two produce a total of four; and so on. It takes a great deal of good food to enable this cell division to take place, and so I believe that the pregnancy diet becomes especially important from the third to sixth month of gestation.

By the end of the sixth month of pregnancy, most of Jimmy's cell division is over. In other words, Jimmy will have as many individual brain cells as he'll ever have in his life by the end of the sixth month of your pregnancy.

You may have heard that adults can destroy brain cells through alcohol or other means and that these cells can never be replaced. And it's absolutely true that lost adult brain cells can't be recovered. But it's also been true since that sixth month you spent in your mother's womb.

It is not clear what effect, if any, the loss of some of the millions of a person's brain cells has upon mental functioning. Some scientists think the loss of a few cells does not make much difference. But I prefer to play it safe. In my judgment, it is best to try to keep and nourish all the brain cells you can at every stage of life, and especially during the early, formative years. Too little is known now about what subtle intellectual skills may depend on certain parts of this vast, intricate human computer we call the brain.

So I would suggest that when you become pregnant, you take as few chances as possible of damaging your unborn child's mental capacities in this important stage of development. Pay especially close attention to your pregnancy diet from the second trimester on, when your child's brain cells are winding up their process of division. A sample one-week diet, which will cover all your unborn child's brain-growth needs, is included in the following chapter.

Jimmy's Brain from the Final Stage of Pregnancy Through Age Five: Cell Development

This exciting phase of Jimmy's brain growth begins around the seventh month of your pregnancy (or the thirty-second week) and ends anywhere from three to five years after birth, depending on which authority one consults. The major part of this stage is the so-called brain growth spurt, which involves rapid expansion of the brain's physical structure up to about age three. What you eat during the last months of your pregnancy and what you feed your child during the first five years after his birth is *absolutely crucial* in determining his later mental potential.

The dramatic nature of this fast growth can be understood better if you consider the increase in the size of your son's brain in terms of percentages: At birth, his brain has reached about 25 percent of its adult weight. By one year, it's up to about 70 percent. And by age three, Jimmy's brain will have increased to approximately 80 percent of its eventual adult size.

If you could open a "window" in Jimmy's head during this period and then magnify his brain many times, you'd be able to observe three "main events" taking place—almost like the featured show in each ring of a three-ring circus. Each main event is very important in determining his later mental capacity. Here they are:

Main Event Number 1: In this first "event," Jimmy's brain cells begin to branch out. Remember how in the second stage of your youngster's brain growth, the cells divide and increase in number? Now, they shoot out little "fingers," or structures call *dendrites* and *spines*. These branches go back and forth between the cells, intertwine with one another, and establish the important connections (called *synapses*) between brain cells.

After these connections are complete, a nerve impulse or message can travel from one cell body down an axon (the brain cell's "extension cord"); to a dendrite (or "branch"); across a synapse (or inter-cell connection);

and finally into the next cell structure. Jimmy can now begin to think!

All this may sound rather simple, as though what happens is like plugging one of your living room lamps into a wall socket. But believe me, it isn't. Some thirty different chemical substances—called "neurotransmitters"—are now known to help transmit nerve impulses from one of Jimmy's brain cells to the next. "Messages" that go across the synapses alone involve an unbelievably elaborate sequence of molecular events. In fact, if you were somehow able to follow all the movements and interactions in your son's head with separate tracers of light, you'd find yourself viewing the most incredible fireworks display imaginable.

The point of all this is that most scientists believe that Jimmy's intelligence is directly related to the branching out of his brain cells and the quality of the connections, or synapses, which they form with one another. In other words, the more efficiently nerve impulses move around in his brain, the better he can think. Naturally, the stronger the physical foundation that you can help lay for the transmittal of these messages and signals in your child's brain, the more intelligent he is likely to be.

As far as we can tell at this point, the way this physical foundation is established in the preschool child is through a interaction of three factors: (1) heredity; (2) environment, including early parental encouragement and education; and (3) good nutrition.

Of course, none of this has been proven beyond the shadow of a doubt. But all indications suggest that these are the most important sources of maximum intellectual development. So you should keep all three of these factors in mind and do everything possible to maximize their presence in the development of your preschool youngster.

Main Event Number 2: The second major thing that happens during Jimmy's cell development phase, as he moves through infancy to toddlerhood, is the *multiplication of supporting cells* in his brain. These are called *glial* cells, and they are composed mainly of fats and cholesterol. Their primary function is to provide a special kind of filter that protects his brain.

You see, Jimmy's brain cells are extremely sensitive to poisonous substances—so much so that a special filter system is needed to keep harmful substances out. This filter protector, known as the "blood-brain barrier," is effective because of two key features: the thickness of the blood vessels in the brain; and the presence of the tight sheaths of supporting (glial) cells around the blood vessels.

So, if the supporting cells in Jimmy's brain grow and multiply properly during this third phase of his brain growth, the protective filtration system will be in a better position to protect the brain—and permit it to develop to its full potential. It is essential, then, that you, as a parent concerned with your child's mind, create an environment in which his brain will have the greatest chance to grow. And one of the most important things about any aspect of a child's physical development—including the growth of his brain—is proper food. That's what *The Brain Food Diet for Children* is all about: It's a practical guide to help you provide your child with the nutritional requirements for healthy brain growth.

Main Event Number 3: There is one other event in the mental "three-ring circus" that occurs during Jimmy's final stage of brain growth. This is another protective process called "myelination," which involves the formation of a protective sheath around each of his brain cells and continues up until he is four or five years old.

As the supporting (glial) cells form a protective armor around the blood vessels in Jimmy's brain (see above), they also proceed to surround each brain cell. While the glial cells are multiplying during Jimmy's earliest years, they also curve around each brain cell in a spiral fashion. After this "wrapping" process is over, Jimmy's body—which should be receiving plenty of fats through his diet—deposits fats and lipids, such as cholesterol, between the supporting (glial) cells and the brain cells (neurons). These deposits form what we call the *myelin*, or protective sheath around each cell.

This protective sheath serves as a kind of insulation for each brain cell and eventually covers each and every cell. The entire process probably lasts until Jimmy is about five years old. If sheaths are damaged or destroyed, Jimmy may contract some disease or suffer brain impairment.

One interesting theory about the function of these sheaths is that they enhance coordination in infants and preschoolers. You've undoubtedly noticed that toddlers at age two or so can't do certain physical tasks as well as older children and adults. For example, they can't control their bodies in sophisticated ways, catch balls with aplomb, or manipulate forks and spoons easily.

As a child gets older and approaches school age, however, the ability to engage in fine muscle-motor activity and advanced feats of physical coordination increases. The increase in such skills corresponds with the youngster's advancing myelination, or formation of protective sheaths around the brain cells. In other words, Jimmy may have passed through his "growth spurt" stage of brain expansion by the time he is three. But before his brain can reach its full physical capacity, he must still undergo that all-important cell-sheathing process which happens up to about age five.

So, to summarize, what we have happening during this third and final phase of Jimmy's brain growth, is that his brain cells grow and extend, and the supporting cells and protective sheaths grow and extend right along with them. Moreover, these physical and biochemical developments, taken together, are probably directly related to Jimmy's potential intelligence. They are the physical base from which he will be able to assimilate new information, process it, and apply it to achieve his goals later in life.

At birth, Jimmy's brain cell development is only about one-sixth completed. Thus the majority of his brain expansion will occur in the early years just after birth—the years during which you must assume responsibility for feeding him properly. I believe following *The Brain Food Diet for Children* is the best way to accomplish the goal of good nutrition for the mind.

Now, pause for a moment and reflect on some of the nutritional implications of your child's pattern of brain growth. While the brain is still developing during the "brain growth spurt" from the seventh month of pregnancy until about age three, there's still time to correct inadequate nutrition. The brain cells, the supporting cells, and the protective sheaths are still multiplying, extending, and connecting. During this period of your youngster's development, good brain food can help establish a physical foundation that will enhance her brain power for the rest of her life. But once the brain spurt is over, after about age four or five, any damage that has occurred in those early years from poor nutrition becomes part of her mental equipment for life.

So, in practical terms, what can you do to ensure that

your child has the best chance to develop her maximum brain power?

To answer this question, let's start with the proper program for your child's brain growth during your pregnancy.

4

How to Feed Your Child Brain Food Before Birth

How important is good nutrition during pregnancy in enhancing your child's potential brain power?

As we've seen already, damage done to a child's brain during pregnancy from malnutrition—as long as it's not severe—can *probably* be reversed since only a small portion of the brain's growth spurt occurs in the womb. But I prefer to play it safe and recommend good nutrition at *all* times during the child's life, including those last couple of months inside the mother. And of course, this means that it's essential for the pregnant woman to pay close attention to her diet. Listen to what another doctor has to say on this subject.

"There is evidence that maternal nutritional status before and during pregnancy influences fetal birth weight and brain development," writes Dr. Kamran S. Moghissi in *Nutritional Impacts on Women*. "Therefore, excessive dietary restrictions in pregnancy are ill advised. The lack of certain amino acids in the diet of pregnant women may have deleterious effect[s]. Furthermore, the quality of ingested food during gestation may exert important effects on the functional ability of the brain in later life."

In other words, even though there is evidence that malnutrition during pregnancy can be corrected, we should not forget that at birth the brain weighs 25 percent of its eventual adult weight. In short, it is important to pay close attention to that crucial first 25 percent! Also, remember the brain is one-sixth of the way through its brain growth spurt at birth. So, it's advisable to get off to a good start during the initial one-sixth of the spurt— and not force your child into the position of playing "catch-up" during the next four to five years.

At the very least, then, pregnancy provides an excellent opportunity to establish a pattern of healthy brain growth. With this principle in mind, what can a woman do to encourage her child's proper brain development during pregnancy?

In general, I recommend three things: (1) maintain your ideal weight before pregnancy; (2) eat at least enough for *one* during pregnancy; and (3) eat high energy foods. Now, let's discuss each of these three "pregnancy principles" in some detail before we consider the specific foods a prospective mother should be eating.

Pregnancy Principle Number 1:
Maintain Your Ideal Weight
Before Pregnancy

Many women start thinking in terms of watching their diet after they conceive. But actually, it's important to get in shape—especially in terms of your nutritional balance—*before* you become pregnant. If you're under-nourished in some way at the time you conceive, then you'll find you have to eat more to nourish yourself and your growing baby. But if you're taking in the right foods when you get pregnant, both you and your unborn baby will be able to make the transition through pregnancy and birth more smoothly and in better health.

Pregnancy Principle Number 2:
Eat at Least Enough for One
After You Become Pregnant

What surprises a lot of people is that mothers-to-be who are really healthy don't appear to have to increase their dietary intake significantly at any stage of pregnancy.

But how, you may ask, can the fetal, the placental, and the various maternal tissues that are necessary during pregnancy be built up without extra food being taken in by the prospective mother?

Researcher Dr. John Dobbing of the University of Manchester Medical School in England says the answer is an increased dietary efficiency on the part of the mother. In the first part of pregnancy, stores of fat are laid down and dietary protein is retained. Then, in the next phase, the fat and protein stores are donated to the developing maternal and fetal tissues. In other words, these new "pregnancy tissues" result not from increased intake, but from decreased excretion. Dobbing says a twofold benefit is the result: (1) "the normal mother [is] relieved of the need to eat more during pregnancy, and (2) "she will not increase the rate of growth of her fetus even if she does."

Remember, though, that these observations don't apply to the improperly nourished mother. She should probably eat enough for two and may need some sort of nutritional supplementation for normal growth of her fetus. As a practical matter, many women in our society need to eat extra food during their pregnancy because they are too thin before conception. So, if you're underweight according to your doctor's evaluation or according to charts that present your ideal weight according to your height and body type, by all means, eat for two!

Medical research suggests that the minimum number of calories you should eat during pregnancy to avoid retarding fetal growth is 1,500 to 1,800 calories per day. To be on the safe side—especially for women who are overly thin when they become pregnant—many doctors now recommend 2,600 to 2,800 calories daily.

Pregnancy Principle Number 3:
Eat High Energy Foods

There was a time not too long ago when extra proteins were thought to be necessary for fetal growth, including the proper development of the unborn child's brain. For one thing, proteins make up a large portion of the brain, and so some people naturally assumed that the pregnant woman should increase her protein intake. As it turns out, though, things don't work quite that way.

In one research study reported in 1980 in New York and interpreted by Dr. John Dobbing of the University of Manchester in an editorial in *Early Human Development*, researchers found no enhancement of fetal growth when pregnant women bolstered their diets with protein-rich supplements. In fact, there were even some indications of harm associated with raised protein intake because more babies were born prematurely, with more serious consequences.

But while excessive amounts of protein are not advisable during pregnancy, foods that *are* appropriate are high-energy complex carbohydrates. These foods, which include such things as vegetables and fruits, contain much more immediately usable energy than proteins.

It has been estimated that the pregnant mother, especially in the last weeks of pregnancy, must supply an extra 300 calories of energy foods (i.e., complex carbohydrates) daily just for her own body's use. One reason is that the growing fetus demands up to 300 calories daily from the mother's body in the last weeks of gestation. Also, the mother requires extra energy for the synthesis of protein in the placenta, for the various maternal membranes, the enlarged uterus, the mammary glands, and the extra fat that always accumulates on the prospective mother's frame.

If you are eating enough food before you become pregnant to meet these extra needs, then you don't need to increase the intake of complex carbohydrates. In other words, if you're eating in the upper range of calories mentioned above (2,600 to 2,800 calories per day), you're probably taking in more than an adequate amount of food for yourself and your baby. But remember: You should always check any pregnancy diet with your doctor.

Now, here is a sample weekly diet for a typical pregnant woman, which was formulated with the foregoing principles in mind. Daily consumption is set at about 2200-plus calories. In choosing this calorie range, I have made two basic assumptions: (1) The pregnant woman is not exceptionally thin (in which case she would need more food); and (2) most women would prefer to play it safe at a calorie level somewhat higher than the minimum of 1500 to 1800 calories.

PREGNANCY DIET: Day 1

Breakfast:
  ½ cup orange juice
  ½ cup oatmeal
  1 whole wheat biscuit
  1 teaspoon margarine
  8 oz. milk

Lunch:
  1½ cups green pea soup
  ½ cup cabbage and carrot slaw
  1 slice oatmeal bread or muffin
  1 teaspoon margarine
  4 oz. milk

Supper:
  3 oz. smothered steak with mushrooms and tomatoes
  ½ cup enriched brown rice
  BAKED PUMPKIN:
  RECIPE: Dice it, then bake at 375°F for 20 to 25 minutes, or boil
  it for 15 to 20 minutes.
      Lettuce, cucumber, and tomato salad
  1 teaspoon oil and vinegar dressing
  1 whole wheat roll
  1 pat butter
  8 oz. milk

Two snacks, served anytime:
  (1)   Peanut butter and grilled cheese sandwich, using 1
             slice whole wheat or rye bread
      4 oz. milk
  (2) 1 oz. Cheddar cheese
  ORANGE AND APPLE COCKTAIL:
  RECIPE: Use ½ small orange and ½ small apple. Wash apple and
  orange, and dice them. Pour lemon juice over the diced fruit
  and mix. Serve in a fruit cocktail glass. 3½-ounce serving.

PREGNANCY DIET: Day 2

Breakfast:
>   ½ cup tomato juice
>   1 deviled egg
>   2 slices whole bran toast
>   1 teaspoon margarine
>   8 oz. milk

Lunch:
>   1 cup black beans, cooked with grated cheese
>   Mixed green salad
>   1 teaspoon Italian dressing
>   1 piece corn bread, 2 inches by 2 inches
>   1 teaspoon margarine or butter
>   8 oz. milk

Supper:
>   3 oz. lamb-on-skewers
>   1 medium baked potato
>   ½ cup broccoli
>   ½ cup sour cooked beets
>   1 whole wheat roll
>   1 pat margarine or butter
>   8 oz. milk

Two snacks, served any time:
>   (1)   4 oz. plain yogurt
>   ¼ cup red berries
>   (2)   1 apple
>   8 oz. milk

PREGNANCY DIET: Day 3

Breakfast:
>½ cup orange juice
>½ cup cooked cereal, or ¾ cup bran flakes
>1 slice whole wheat grain toast
>1 pat margarine
>8 oz. milk

Lunch:
>Sandwich: 2 oz. turkey on whole grain bread
>1 pat margarine

>RAINBOW SALAD:
>RECIPE: Mix ½ cup watermelon and cantaloupe balls with 1½ teaspoons chopped raisins, then stir in 3 small powdered walnuts. Pour ½ teaspoon lemon juice over mixture before serving.
>8 oz. milk

Supper:
>2 oz. meat loaf
>½ cup mashed potatoes, or 1 medium baked potato
>½ cup carrot rings
>½ cup cabbage slaw
>1 apple
>1 slice enriched whole grain roll
>1 pat margarine
>8 oz. milk

Two snacks, served any time:
>(1) 1 slice enriched whole grain or rye bread
>   1 oz. Cheddar cheese
>   8 oz. any natural fruit juice
>(2) 8 oz. milk
>   1 peanut butter cookie

PREGNANCY DIET: Day 4

Breakfast:
- ½ cup orange juice
- ¾ cup bran cereal
- 1 soya muffin
- 1 pat margarine
- 8 oz. milk

Lunch:

TUNA AND CHEESE "MELT":

RECIPE: Use ¼ cup tuna, 1 oz. Cheddar cheese, 1 medium tomato, 1 slice cracked wheat bread. Put tuna, sliced tomato, and Cheddar cheese on top of bread. Place in oven and heat until cheese melts.

Supper:

CHICKEN SUPREME:

RECIPE: Use 2 oz. boned chicken, 1 egg, ¼ cup milk, ¼ cup celery, salt and pepper to taste. Cut the chicken and celery in squares. Add to slightly beaten egg. Add milk, pepper, and salt. Place mixture in a mold, set in a pan of water, and bake until firm at 345°. Turn out onto a plate and serve.
- ½ cup summer salad
- 1 small piece corn bread
- 1 pat margarine
- 8 oz. milk

Two snacks, served any time:
- (1) 1 cup spinach soup
       1 slice whole wheat bread, or 2 whole grain crackers
       ½ cup carrot and cabbage slaw
       4 oz. milk
- (2) 8 oz. milk

STRAWBERRY AND MINT PEAR:

RECIPE: Use ½ ripe pear, ½ cup strawberries, 2 mint sprigs, lettuce. Wash pear thoroughly and cut in two. Chop mint leaves after washing. Roll the pear halves in the mint leaves. Set the pear on a lettuce leaf, and fill the center with strawberries. Decorate sides of pears with extra strawberries. Serve chilled.

PREGNANCY DIET: Day 5

Breakfast:
- ½ cup grapefruit sections
- ½ cup oatmeal
  Banana bran muffin
- 1 pat margarine
- 8 oz. milk

Lunch:
- 1 cup lima beans, cooked with grated cheese
  Rainbow salad
- 1 tablespoon Italian dressing
- 1 oatmeal cookie
- 8 oz. milk

Supper:
- Walnut omelet (ordinary omelet, with filling of chopped walnuts)
- 1 medium baked potato
  Carrot and cabbage slaw
- 2 plums
- 8 oz. milk

Two snacks, served any time:
- (1) 2 slices whole wheat bread
      2 tablespoons peanut butter
      4 oz. milk
- (2) Sandwich: 2 oz. turkey with mayonnaise, on 2 slices of enriched bread
      1 cucumber
      4 oz. milk

PREGNANCY DIET: Day 6

Breakfast:
- ½ cup orange juice
- 1 scrambled egg
- 1 whole wheat muffin
- 1 teaspoon margarine
- 8 oz. milk

Lunch:
- 1½ cups split pea soup
- Mixed vegetable salad
- 1 slice whole wheat bread
- 1 teaspoon margarine
- 8 oz. milk

Supper:
- 3 oz. broiled ground beef
- 1 medium baked potato
- Tomato, lettuce, and cucumber salad
- 1 tablespoon oil and vinegar dressing
- 1 slice whole wheat bread
- 1 teaspoon margarine
- 8 oz. milk

Two snacks, served any time:
- (1) 1 tablespoon peanut butter served on 1 slice rye bread
  - 1 oz. hard cheese
  - 1 cup orange and pineapple juice cocktail
- (2) 1 small apple
  - 1 oz. Cheddar cheese

PREGNANCY DIET: Day 7

Breakfast:
- ½ cup melon
- 1 slice whole wheat banana bread
- 2 tablespoons peanut butter
- 8 oz. milk

Lunch:
- 2 oz. Cheddar cheese
- 1 slice whole wheat bread
  Salad of tomatoes, lettuce, onions, and mushrooms
- 1 cup yogurt, topped by raisins and slivered almonds
- 8 oz. pineapple juice

Supper:
- 4 oz. broiled steak
- 1 cup brown rice with 2 tablespoons margarine
- 1 cup stewed cabbage and carrots
- 4 oz. milk

Two snacks, served any time:
- (1) 1 slice angel food cake
       ½ cup sliced strawberries and pear
       4 oz. milk
- (2) 8 oz. milk
       1 apple
       1 oz. Cheddar cheese
       2 bread sticks

With menus like these each day during pregnancy, you'll be able to keep yourself healthy. And most important of all, you'll give your unborn child an excellent start toward achieving his ultimate intellectual potential.

But this is only the first step. Now, let's consider the most effective diet plan to nourish the brain power of your youngster from birth to age five.

5

The Mother's Milk Principle

Since the beginning of recorded history, great importance has been placed on the nursing of children by their mothers. In fact, in earlier times (and also in undeveloped societies today) children were fed at the mother's breasts until they were at least two or three years old. It goes without saying that this is a much older age than we usually tolerate in our own fast-moving society, where mothers tend to feel tied down by a suckling toddler.

Of course, one of the reasons for the popularity of breast-feeding is that mother's milk has always been a ready and inexpensive source of nourishment for the young. But more than that, it's the most natural and time-honored means to give a youngster the best start in life. In fact, in earlier days, other important activities or objectives for the child were commonly postponed until the "suckling" stage had been completed.

For example, the Hebrew prophet Samuel was dedicated by his mother Hannah to God, and she turned him over to the priest Eli at a very young age—but *only* after he had been weaned. According to the Bible, Samuel immediately started "ministering to the Lord" when he was given to Eli, and so he must have been old enough to get about by himself, understand the priest, and respond to commands. (1 Sam. 1:21–24; 2:11.) From what I know about the relative abilities of young children from my own practice, I'd say he would have had to be at least three or four years old at the time that he finished breast-feeding and joined the priest Eli.

This tradition is revealed again in the apocryphal Hebrew book of the Maccabees (2 Macc. 7:27–28), where a mother urges her son to flout the evil King Antiochus by reminding him, "My son, take pity on me. I carried you nine months in the womb, suckled you three years, reared you and brought you up to your present age."

Nor is the extended nursing concept limited to the Judeo-Christian tradition. In Islam, there is a rule in feeding young children that says, "Mothers shall give suck to their children twofold years."

Historical studies have revealed no significant practice of artificial feeding of infants and young toddlers before the seventeenth century. When the forerunners of the modern liquid formulas for babies did appear, they could not measure up to the real substance from the mother's breast. Even today, no formula can compare with mother's milk, either for a baby's general dietary needs or for the specific requirements of the child's growing brain. In fact, it's impossible to find any single sort of food that is the nutritional equal of breast-feeding for children up to three years of age.

For these reasons, I advocate what I call the "Mother's Milk Principle" of nutrition for the best brain development of young children. In short, the basic principle may be stated this way: For at least the first three years of life—and in a modified form up to age five—the proportions of carbohydrates, fats, and proteins in the diet of a young child should come as close as possible to those of breast milk. This means that fats in the child's daily calorie consumption should range up to 50 percent; complex carbohydrates should be 35 to 45 percent; and the proteins in his diet should be 8 to 15 percent.

Now, there's nothing at all radical about this concept. In fact, in 1979, the Committee on Nutrition of the American Academy of Pediatrics said, "Breast milk has not been improved upon as a reference standard [for a young child's nutrition]." Despite the fact that corporations have spent millions trying to find a formula to surpass breast milk's nutritional quality, the mother still does the best job and probably always will.

But as a practical matter, most mothers in our society either can't or won't nurse their children much past one year of age, and the outside limit is usually five or six months. So, the use of formula, and solid foods in the right proportions becomes a necessity—especially as far as the development of the child's brain is concerned. And here's where the Mother's Milk Principle comes in.

As we have seen, the distribution of calories in a child's diet up to about age five should conform generally with the distribution of percentages of fat calories, carbohydrate calories, and protein calories in healthy breast milk. Of course, as we'll see later, there is an acceptable range of flexibility for these percentages that varies up and down a few percentage points. But in general, these values reflect what modern medical studies show to be the best brain food diet—and the best program for overall nutrition as well.

Some parents who look at these percentages may exclaim, "But the fats are so high! What about cholesterol and the advice we hear about keeping fatty foods low?"

And you're absolutely right: The fat content of this diet *is* high in comparison with a healthy diet for most adults. In fact, many nutrition experts *reverse* the fat and carbohydrate distribution I have proposed for preschool children. They feel that calories in the daily adult diet should be composed of 50 percent complex carbohydrates; 30 percent fats; and 20 percent proteins.

But for children the important thing to keep in mind is that mother's milk is very high in fats—indeed, as high as I am suggesting in *The Brain Food Diet for Children!* Studies of the composition of human milk show that it contains about 55 percent fats, 37 percent carbohydrates, and 8 percent proteins.

Now, it's true that some physicians have expressed concern that atherosclerosis, or hardening of the arteries from too high a fat content in the blood, may begin at a relatively young age. But there have been no studies that show there is any danger of feeding very young children fats in accordance with the Mother's Milk Principle. The fact is, a child needs more fats in her diet than an adult, at least up to age three and probably up to age five—largely because of the tremendous brain development that takes place during this time of life.

This need for a relatively high proportion of fats in the child's diet is a theme which runs through much medical literature—and is also perhaps the most important theme in this book. My advice to parents would be: Don't feed your preschooler an adult diet that is low in fats. Rather, if you want to maximize your chances of increasing your child's brain power, *follow the Mother's Milk Principle and keep the distribution of fats up around 50 percent.* (But of course, if your family has a history of high blood lipid levels, you should consult your physician before putting your child on this high-fat brain food diet.)

To understand the Mother's Milk Principle more fully, it is helpful to think back on our discussion about brain growth and development during the preschool years. At birth the baby's brain has completed only one-sixth of its brain-growth spurt. In other words, the large majority of this spurt lies ahead, in the first three years of life.

This spurt includes the formation of the brain's supporting cells, the laying down of the protective sheaths around each cell, and the branching out of each individual brain cell. Then, from age three to five, the brain continues to grow more slowly, and the all-important process of myelination (or covering of brain cells with sheaths) proceeds to completion.

In the opinion of many physicians and scientists, all these developments are essential in establishing the physical basis for a person's intelligence. Naturally, it takes an intake of certain materials—specific foods and fuels—to complete such a job. And it just so happens that mother's milk has all the right materials, in the right proportions, to encourage the proper physical development of the brain.

In fact, in one recent study, Dr. Shirley P. Misa of the Memorial Hospital Medical Center of Long Beach, California, discovered this interesting fact, reported in *Pediatric News:* "Very-low-birthweight infants [who are] fed their mother's breast milk have more rapid growth of head circumference in relation to their weight during the first few weeks of life than their peers [who are] fed high-calorie formulas." Of course, as we've seen, there's no decisive evidence that high intelligence is connected with relatively large head circumference. But a healthy head size is at least one indication that things are going well in the brain area.

To help us understand more clearly the rationale

behind the Mother's Milk Principle, let's take a closer look at the major components of breast milk.

Component Number One: Water About 88 percent of most breast milk is made up of water.

Component Number Two: Fats While fats provide the majority of the calories in breast milk, they also are breast milk's most variable component. On average, breast milk is about 3.8 percent fat, though one nursing mother's fat content may vary anywhere from 2.0 to 6.0 percent. The highest concentration of fat measured in one study was nearly 11 percent of the total content of the breast milk!

Part of this variation is due to the quality of the mother's food intake, and part is due to the time during nursing when the milk is tested. You see, the first flow of milk drawn from the breast (called the *foremilk*) may contain only 1 percent fat. In contrast, milk at the end of a nursing session (the *hindmilk*) may contain as much as 7 to 8 percent fat.

This variance is normal, and scientists now believe that the high fat content during the last part of a nursing session has a healthy "satiating effect" on the infant's appetite. That is, the infant gets "filled up" after he has received the many non-fat nutrients, but before the bulk of the fat comes into the milk flow. As a result, he stops eating before he consumes too many calories.

Some scientists have even gone so far as to suggest that since bottled formula does not and cannot vary the fat content of a single feeding, the baby on a bottle often can't learn in a natural way when to stop feeding. Consequently, he may take in too many fatty calories, and the stage may be set for obesity in later life. Other experts, though, counter this view by pointing to some pudgy breast-fed babies who, in many cases, may be heavier than those fed by bottle.

Whatever the merits of these arguments, the fact remains that the nutrients in the varying fat content of breast milk are extremely important for the brain development of the young child. Scientists have found, for example, that the levels of two major fats intimately associated with brain development (the arachidonic and decosahexaenoic acids) are ten times higher in human milk than in cow's milk. While it is possible to some extent for the infant to manufacture these essential fats from cow's milk, human milk makes things much easier for the baby's physical system.

Cholesterol, too, is another fat present in high levels in breast milk. Despite the bad publicity that this fatty substance has received for its role in causing hardening of the arteries in adults, cholesterol is absolutely essential for the proper brain growth of the young child.

As has been mentioned, some experts believe young children who take in too much cholesterol may develop the beginnings of atherosclerosis, or hardening of the arteries. But there is another strong line of opinion that says giving a child significant amounts of cholesterol will help his body process it better later—and will thereby protect him in his adult years against atherosclerosis.

So the atherosclerosis issue is very much up in the air right now. As for myself, I'm convinced that the need of the growing brain for fats and cholesterol, especially up to age three, far outweighs any unsubstantiated fears about hardening of the arteries much later in adult life.

So what exactly will cholesterol do for your child's brain? Specifically, cholesterol is an important ingredient in at least two brain-growth processes:

• The biochemical development of the brain:

Remember in the final brain development stage (myelination) how lipids wrap around the brain cells to form a protective sheath? The lipids include cholesterol, and that's why it's so vital to have sufficient cholesterol present for proper brain development.

- **The manufacturing of "enzymatic systems":** Enzymes are special compounds that help stimulate chemical reactions in the body. They keep the internal chemicals in the body "moving," and without them, we simply couldn't live. Since cholesterol is involved in manufacturing these enzymes, it's obviously an essential ingredient in the child's mental and physical well-being.

In conclusion, my point here is simple: While adults should curb their intake of cholesterol, infants definitely should not. Cholesterol is required for proper brain development, and breast milk is the best available source.

Component Number Three: Protein This third major component of breast milk, protein, usually comprises between 1.0 and 1.4 percent of the mother's flow. This percentage may seem low in comparison with cow's milk (which has 3.3 percent protein) or some of today's formulas. And it is low—with good reason!

You see, many scientists no longer consider protein to be the darling of infant nutrition. The fact is, newborn infants who are given high protein formulas, may in some instances develop a condition called *transient neonatal tyrosenimia,* which is believed to cause some mental impairment. Similarly, it has been suggested that the absence of two key amino acids (taurine and cystine) in certain protein-rich formulas may also negatively affect brain development.

Breast milk, in contrast, appears to have *all* the right proteins, in the proper proportions, for successful brain development. In fact, you will even find two anti-infective proteins in breast milk—lysizyme and lactoferrin—which help protect your newborn baby against disease. This is an important point in proper brain development because an ill infant usually doesn't eat properly. If a baby gets very sick, she may even become somewhat dehydrated and malnourished. These conditions, especially if they recur regularly or if they continue on one occasion for a relatively long period of time, can present a threat to healthy brain growth.

Component Number Four: Carbohydrates Carbohydrates in the diets of both children and adults are high-energy foods that serve as the main "fuel" for daily life. They supply calories that can be easily processed to keep our internal body functions and our external activities going at full tilt. Lactose, a simple sugar, which is "in solution" (or dissolved) in mother's milk, is the major carbohydrate in breast food; it comprises from about 6.6 to 8.0 percent of the total substance.

Unlike some other nutrients, lactose varies only slightly when you compare well-nourished women with those who are undernourished. Maternal diet seems to have little effect on the carbohydrate content of breast milk.

Component Number Five: Vitamins and minerals Unlike carbohydrates, the vitamin and mineral content of breast milk is strongly influenced by the mother's diet. So, if the mother is malnourished, breast feeding will not be sufficient, and some sort of supplementation will be in order.

In terms of brain development, there is no known

"wonder vitamin" or "super mineral" that can enhance intelligence. But breast milk from well-nourished women does seem to have all the right vitamins and minerals in the proper proportions to ensure healthy development of the entire body, including the brain.

For example, for years scientists thought breast milk was inadequate in Vitamin D. But rickets, a disease caused by Vitamin D deficiency, is rarely found in breast-fed infants. In other words, in some way youngsters on mother's milk seem to be getting enough Vitamin D.*

The same principle applies to iron. While the absolute concentration of this mineral in breast milk is low, few breast-fed infants exhibit iron deficiency.

Is there a reason for these seeming paradoxes?

What appears to be happening is that the nutrients in breast milk are more easily absorbed by the infant. As a result, less of these nutrients are required. Doctors call this phenomenon *improved bioavailability*. That is, the child's body can absorb various nutrients more easily because other facilitating substances in breast milk assist the youngster's system in food processing.

These five components, then, are the main ingredients of breast milk. But there are other "trace substances"—or nutrients in small amounts—which may be of potential benefit to the brain of your child. These include various enzymes and hormones, but even today not too much is known about the role they play in our physical development. Still, there are some positive indi-

---

NOTE: Even though most breast-feeding children seem to get enough Vitamin D, I still recommend Vitamin D supplements for them, just to be on the safe side.

cations that breast milk is important in ways we can't yet comprehend.

So, while formulas may try to copy mother's milk—and they can succeed to a certain degree—there are features of breast milk that formulas simply can't duplicate. These unique qualities of breast milk include:

- The interplay between different constituents of breast milk that enhances absorption of nutrients;
- The "just-right" proportions of all the components of breast milk;
- The variation in percentage of fat from start to finish of a single feeding; and
- The all-important interaction that occurs between mother and child as the infant feeds at the breast.

This last feature, by the way, is often called "bonding." Bonding is such an important concept in promoting a child's maximum potential intelligence, that I want to devote some space to explaining what it's all about.

The term comes from the special bond, formed through such factors as physical closeness and eye contact, which develops between the mother and child during breast-feeding. Even though there isn't a direct connection that can be identified between the quality of bonding and the level of brain power, there is good reason to believe there are at least important indirect connections.

Let me explain: Some Swedish mothers were tested in 1977 in an effort to determine the impact of bonding. The women, who spent only an additional fifteen minutes of close contact, including suckling, with their babies in the first half hour of life, spent more time looking at the infants and kissing them at three months of age. In contrast, the other mothers, who had not devoted that extra fifteen minutes, spent more time cleaning their babies. Also, the babies of the first group of mothers cried significantly less and smiled significantly more than the children of the other mothers.

The point here is that the very early bond that is formed between mother and child during breast-feeding—even when that bond involves just a few minutes of the mother's time—is extremely important to the child's later behavior and emotional development. And of course, if a child feels secure, positive, and emotionally stable, he is likely to be in a position to make the best use of the brain power he has.

In my opinion, then—for a variety of reasons—"breast is best" for a child's intellectual development. Without any hesitation, I strongly recommend breast-feeding at least for the first four to six months after the birth of your child.

But now, what about the foods that a breast-feeding mother should be consuming to be sure that her milk is up to par?

You may be surprised at how little your food intake needs to increase during lactation. It is only a matter of about 500 calories per day over the normal diet for your height and weight. The reason is that the mother's body has been preparing for lactation all during pregnancy and has built up a "fat bank," if you will, to be used for milk production.

But even though your food intake needs to go up by 500 calories, it's important to be sure that you're getting the proper daily allowances of key vitamins, minerals, and other nutrients. The main ones are listed below:

Energy (kcal)	2600
Protein (g)	66
Vitamin A (IU)	6000

Vitamin D (IU)	400
Vitamin E (IU)	15
Vitamin C (IU)	100
Folacin (ug)	500
Niacin (mg)	18
Riboflavin (mg)	1.8
Thiamine (mg)	1.5
Vitamin B_6 (mg)	2.5
Vitamin B_{12} (ug)	4.0
Calcium (mg)	1200
Phosphorus (mg)	1200
Iodine (ug)	200
Iron* (mg)	18
Magnesium (mg)	450
Zinc (mg)	25

Now, let's say you did all the right things during and after pregnancy: You ate all the right foods, and you're in the process of breast-feeding. You can feel satisfied that you've gotten your child off to the best start possible in his journey toward his maximum intelligence. But this is no time to become complacent. Next comes the most difficult, and perhaps the most important period of all—the experience of getting the youngster on a good brain food diet after breast-feeding.

NOTE: 30-60 mg. additional iron each day for 2-3 months after delivery is advisable to replenish the iron stores depleted by pregnancy.

6

The Brain Food
Diet from
Birth to Age One

From the time your child is born until he reaches his sixth birthday, what you feed him can be decisive in terms of his brain growth.

Remember: It's during the first three years of life that the "brain growth spurt" occurs. After that, further important brain development, including the "myelination" stage where the cells are sheathed in fatty substances, continues through age four or five. So it's only logical that what you feed your youngster during this important period will be of strategic importance for the physical basis of this later intelligence.

The first natural question that arises is: What kind of food should I feed my child to be sure her brain gets the key nutrients it needs?

To answer this question, I want to focus initially on the child's diet from birth to about one year of age, when solids are being introduced into the diet.

The first section below should be used for the youngster who is breast-feeding, and the second for the child who is formula-fed.*

The dietary needs for a particular child may be determined by first determining the weight of the child. Then you multiply that weight in pounds by a calorie value, which will be indicated for each age group below.

The Breast-Fed Baby, Birth to Age One

Birth to one month old: The child should consume about 55 calories for every pound he weighs, or about 357 to 577 calories a day. (You certainly don't have to worry about making any precise measurement of the calories consumed. If your child is gaining weight and appears satisfied after each feeding, that's enough of an indication that you're doing the right thing.)

There should be approximately eight feedings every day, each about three hours apart. It's best, though, to feed your baby on a "demand" basis—that is, when he's hungry—than on any rigid time schedule. Also, the more you breast-feed your child, the more milk you'll produce. The child should spend ten to twenty minutes at each breast and will consume about 32 ounces of milk daily.

Two months old: The child should consume 50 calories for every pound of weight, or about 475 to 625 calories daily. Eight feedings a day of breast milk, ten to twenty minutes at each breast.

NOTE: The procedure for introducing solids into the diet of a child who is being breast-fed after six months of age is the same as for formula-fed babies and is included under that section.

Three months old: The child should consume 50 calories for every pound of weight, or about 550 to 725 calories daily. Six to eight breast feedings, ten to twenty minutes at each breast.

Four months old: The child should consume 50 calories for every pound of weight, or about 625 to 825 calories per day. Six breast feedings daily, ten to twenty minutes at each breast.

Five months old: The child should consume 50 calories for every pound of weight, or about 675 to 875 calories daily. Five to six breast feedings, ten to twenty minutes at each breast. *Also, begin to introduce solid foods:* Start with 1 to 2 teaspoons of ready-to-serve dry baby cereal (rice, barley, oatmeal, wheat, high-protein, for example) each day; and you may give the child up to 5 to 6 tablespoons daily (1 tablespoon equal 15 calories of protein, carbohydrates and fats). All types of cereal may be introduced, but you should be careful to introduce one at a time, with five days in between each new type. The reason is that it's easier then to recognize allergic reactions to any given type of food.

Six months to one year: At this point many mothers prefer to wean the child, and if so, he should be put on a commercial formula. But if you prefer, it's certainly acceptable—and many physicians believe, desirable—to continue to feed your child by breast, even up to two years of age.

Whatever you decide, though, it's important beginning at this age to introduce the youngster to a complete variety of solid foods offering the different textures, tastes, and ingredients that are necessary for proper growth. On the other hand, it's best not to start the child

on solids at an earlier age, because he may be too immature to refuse foods that are offered, and overfeeding
may result. If you've switched to formula at six months,
continue your child's first-year diet as it is described in
the next section dealing with the formula-fed baby. If
you're still breast feeding, just give your child breast milk
as he desires and follow the formula-fed program for
introducing solids.

As I've said, I strongly favor feeding a baby breast
milk, at least up to six months of age and even older if it's
convenient for the mother. Breast milk has almost all the
right components, in the right proportions, to encourage
proper brain development. The only nutrients you should
supplement during breast-feeding are the following:

Vitamin A: 1500 IU per day (first year of life)
Vitamin C: 35 mg per day (first year)
Vitamin D: 400 IU per day (first year)
Fluoride: 0.25 mg per day (ending at six months to
    one year, depending on the fluoride status of the
    water in your community)

The Formula-Fed Baby, Birth to Age One

Birth to one month old: Each day, the baby should
consume 55 calories multiplied by her weight in pounds,
or about 357 to 577 calories a day. The child should get
six feedings, 3 to 3½ ounces each, of *iron-fortified* formula daily. In general, the commercial formulas have 20
calories per ounce.

Two months old: The child should consume 50 calories multiplied by weight in pounds, or about 475 to 625 calories daily. The child should consume six 3½- to 6-ounce feedings daily.

Three months old: The child should consume 50 calories multiplied by weight in pounds, 550 to 725 calories daily. The child should receive five 4- to 7-ounce feedings daily.

Four months old: The child should consume 50 calories multiplied by weight in pounds, or 625 to 825 calories per day. The child should receive five feedings daily, 5 to 8 ounces at each feeding.

Five months old: The child should consume 50 calories multiplied by weight in pounds, or 675 to 875 calories daily. The child should get five iron-fortified formula feedings each day, with 6 to 8 ounces at each feeding. As with the breast-fed child, solid foods should be introduced beginning at this age. Start with 1 to 2 teaspoons of ready-to-serve dry baby cereal; and you may give your child up to 5 to 6 tablespoons, one to two times a day (1 tablespoon equals 15 calories of protein, carbohydrate, and fat).

Six to eight months old: The child should consume 45 calories multiplied by weight in pounds, or about 788 to 877 calories daily. These calories should consist of about 640 liquid calories (iron-fortified formula or breast milk) and about 147 to 237 calories from solid foods.

My specific recommendation for babies on formula is to serve *five meals a day and limit each serving of a solid to 4 tablespoons.* Foods to serve each day include:

Iron-fortified formula: maximum of 32 ounces daily.

Cereal: 4 to 8 tablespoons daily, or 60 to 120 calories of protein, carbohydrate, and fat.

Vegetables (fresh, finely mashed or bottled baby foods): 8 tablespoons daily equals 48 calories of carbohydrates. (*Caution:* Avoid home-prepared spinach and beets up to one year of age because of the nitrites present in those foods. Cucumbers, cabbage, onions and broccoli are difficult to digest up to age one.)

Fruit (fresh, finely mashed or bottled baby foods): 8 tablespoons daily equals 72 calories of carbohydrates.

Caution: Honey is not recommended as a sweetener during the first year of life because botulism spores may be present in it.

Eight to ten months old: The child should consume 45 calories multiplied by weight in pounds, or 877 to 967 calories daily. As above, meals should be served five times a day, and each serving of a solid should be limited to 4 tablespoons. Liquids (primarily formula) should make up 640 of these calories, and solids 280 to 325. Your child should be drinking a maximum of 32 ounces of formula each day during these two months.

To make up the calories from solids during these months, choose one or more from the following foods. Pay attention to the calorie values, which are listed as numbers in boldface, so that you stay within the 280- to 325-calorie limit each day. The food types—protein, carbohydrate, and fat—are designated by the letters *p, c,* and *f* respectively. Finally, be sure to rotate the food types so that no one food is overemphasized and no one is omitted. Pediatricians like to test the child's reaction to each kind of food to be sure the youngster has no allergic or other negative reaction.

Cereal: 4 tablespoons per day **(60)** *(p,c,f)*
Juice: 3 oz. **(48)** *(c)*
Vegetables: 8 tablespoons **(48)** *(c)*
Fruit: 8 tablespoons **(72)** *(c)*
Meat: 8 tablespoons **(136)** *(p,c,f)*
Fish: ⅛ cup **(40)** *(p,f)*
Yogurt: ¼ cup **(37)** *(p,c,f)*
Cheese: ½ oz. **(56)** *(p,f)*
Dried beans, cooked: ¼ cup **(45)** *(p,c)*
Peanut butter: ½ tablespoon **(43)** *(p,c,f)*
Egg yolk: one **(59)** *(p,f)* Note: Egg white and ice cream which contains egg white should be avoided in the first year because of the potential for allergic reactions.

Ten to twelve months old: The child should consume 45 calories multiplied by weight in pounds, or 967 to 1012 calories daily. These calories should consist of 480 liquid calories and 510 to 530 calories from solid foods. Again, limit each serving of a solid food to 4 tablespoons.

The child should receive about 24 ounces of iron-fortified formula daily at this age.

As for solid foods, choose one or more from the following list. As you choose, keep in mind the principle of rotation of foods and also the principle of staying within the daily solid calorie limits for this age group (510 to 530 calories).*

Cereal: 4 tablespoons **(60)** *(p,c,f)*
Bread: ½ slice **(25)** *(p,c)*
Fruit: 8 tablespoons **(72)** *(c)*

NOTE: Formula-fed children should remain on iron-fortified formula until they are one year old, but no fluoride supplement and no vitamin supplements are needed.

Vegetables: 8 tablespoons (**48**) *(c)*
Yogurt: ½ cup (**75**) *(p,c,f)*
Eggs: 1 whole (**78**) *(p,f)*
Peanut butter: 1 tablespoon (**86**) *(p,c,f)*
Dried beans, cooked: ¼ cup (**45**) *(p,c)*
Meat: 8 tablespoons (**136**) *(p,c,f)*
Fish: 8 tablespoons (**120**) *(p,c,f)*
Chicken: 8 tablespoons (**176**) *(p)*
Juice: 3 oz. (**48**) *(c)*

Now that we've considered what sort of food a baby needs to enhance his maximum brain growth in the first year of life, it's time to move on to the question of how you should feed your child from ages one through five. The components of a mother's milk or of commercial formula provide enough brain food—and especially fats—to do the job in the first year. But most children go off formula or breast milk during the second year of life and begin to eat right along with their parents. The problem is that foods that are healthy for adults are not necessarily the best foods for a child's brain growth. So now let's consider the best way to feed your child's intellect until age five.

7

Feeding the Intellect from One to Five

I n *The Brain Food Diet for Children* I recommend a diet for children age one to five that is virtually the opposite of the usual diet recommended for adults.

The basic principle behind the child's diet, as we've already seen, is this: Children up to age three—and with some modifications through age five—should eat a solid food diet that has approximately the same fat-carbohydrate-protein proportions as breast milk.

The distinctive feature of the children's brain food program is that it's relatively high in fats—just as breast milk is high in fats. To reiterate, the daily percentages of the major food categories that I recommend are: up to 50 percent fats; 35 to 45 percent complex carbohydrates; and 8 to 15 percent protein. The diets in the next few chapters are based on these basic principles and percentages.

More specifically, *The Brain Food Diet for Children* focuses on the following five nutritional elements:

Element Number One: Amino Acids Amino acids are the building blocks of proteins, and they promote general tissue and body growth. In addition, they are vital elements in the proper functioning of the brain and nervous system.

Scientific studies have shown that in animals, for example, "severe protein-calorie malnutrition in early life decreases the number of brain cells and alters the cellular and enzymatic organization of the brain." This information is according to Dr. Merrill S. Read of the National Institute of Child Health and Human Development.

But what do amino acids and proteins actually do when it comes to brain functioning?

If you go back to our earlier description of the brain and nerve cells, you'll find that many amino acids appear to act as "transmitters" for the nervous system. This means that they help transmit nerve impulses from one nerve cell to another. "In fact," says Leslie L. Iversen in *Scientific American*, "the common and abundant amino acids, glutamic acid and aspartic acid, exert powerful . . . effects on most neurons and may well be the commonest [action-producing] transmitters at brain synapses."

This means that amino acids seem to be linked to behavior, learning, and basic intelligence in some way; but their full impact has yet to be completely proven or understood. For example, one thing we do know is that the simplest of all amino acids, called glycine, is an "inhibiting transmitter in the spinal cord," according to Iversen. When found in excess, it may result in lethargy.

So the child's brain does need amino acids. And

while the body can manufacture some of those it needs from other nutrients, nine of them cannot be manufactured. They must come into the body from the outside, in the form of good nutrition. These nine amino acids, which must be supplied through the diet, are called "essential amino acids."

The nine essential amino acids are: histidine, isoleucine, leucine, phenylalanine, methionine, lysine, threonine, tryptophan, and valine. But let me offer one word of caution here: Even though these "essential" amino acids must be supplied from outside the body, it's usually not advisable to try to supplement them through special pills or tablets—at least, not unless your physician prescribes them. In fact, protein supplements have, in some cases, caused physical harm to children.

The protein balance in the human body is rather delicate, and so your child's system will respond better to a good natural diet than to artificial supplements. As long as the youngster is eating 8 to 15 percent of her calories as protein each day, as suggested in the menus in the following chapters, that will be adequate. Foods like eggs, meat, fish, legumes, and whole milk are among the brain foods that supply the essential and other amino acids that the development of a young brain requires.

Element Number Two: Fats As we've already seen, fats and lipids (fatlike substances) are required for the proper physical development of the brain. Specifically, they enter into the formation of the brain's supporting cells, the laying down of the protective sheaths around the brain cells, and the branching out of each individual cell. All of these phases of the brain's growth are now thought to be responsible for a person's potential intelligence level.

In terms of calories, I recommend that your child's fat

intake should vary from about 42 up to 50 percent of the total calories consumed each day. Approximately half of these fats should be saturated and the other half unsaturated.

Unlike a healthy adult diet, cholesterol should be one of the fats which is present in your child's eating program. While it's not certain that dietary cholesterol is used directly to form the nerve and brain cells, protective sheaths, many scientists believe cholesterol is at the very least indirectly involved in the sheaths' formation.

So, fats must be key elements in any diet that centers on brain development. But don't worry about feeding a certain number of grams of cholesterol per day or a certain number of saturated or unsaturated fats per day. If you became involved in such calculations, you'd probably have little time to shop for your child's menus. As long as you follow the dietary program we outline in the following chapters for each age group, you'll achieve the right proportion of fats and cholesterol.

Element Number Three: Water You've probably heard that it's important for a child to drink plenty of liquids. This is quite true. Growing bodies and brains need a lot of water. A lack of sufficient fluids can result in anything from a mildly dehydrated condition and temporarily impaired brain function, to serious, life-threatening convulsions and permanent brain damage.

Of course, these conditions are the extreme. More than likely, children will get enough water to avoid becoming dehydrated as long as they are well. But if they are ill or their environment is excessively warm, they may not have enough water to lubricate their systems properly. Remember: About 88 percent of breast milk is water, and breast milk is the single best brain food we know about!

Here are some guidelines suggesting how much water your preschool child should be taking in each day:

Age	Amount of Water Per Day
Birth to 2½ months	2 to 3 oz. per pound of body weight
2½ months to 8½ months	2 to 2½ oz. per pound
8½ months to 3 years	2 oz. per pound
3 years to 6 years	1½ oz. per pound

From the above chart, you can see that if your child weighs 30 pounds at two years of age, he should have about 60 ounces of water each day. This water, by the way, may come from liquids or solids. For example, foods such as milk, fruits, and vegetables are good sources of water. Even so, you should be very liberal with the amount you encourage your youngster to drink.

Element Number Four: Carbohydrates Complex carbohydrates are necessary in any diet, both to provide bulk for the digestive system and to provide quick energy to enable the person to carry on an active life. As a matter of fact, the brain is especially known for being a high energy user, and so it needs plenty of carbohydrates to function properly.

How many carbohydrates are required?

Approximately 37 percent of the nonwater nutrients in breast milk are carbohydrates, and that's within the range I recommend in *The Brain Food Diet for Children.* Specifically, the diets in this book have been structured so that a child will take in about 35 to 45 percent complex carbohydrates daily.

I should say at this point that I often use the term "complex carbohydrate" rather than simply "carbohydrate," because complex carbohydrates include important foods like fruits and vegetables, while simple carbohydrates encompass the "hollow calories" that are found in sweets and desserts. I *do* recommend the complex carbohydrate group of foods, and those are ones that are included in *The Brain Food Diet for Children*. But I *don't* recommend sugary foods like candy and sweet desserts for children.

Element Number Five: Vitamins and Minerals Vitamins and minerals—especially calcium—must sometimes be supplemented after age one for your child to stay healthy. But in most cases, the youngster's diet can take care of his vitamin and mineral needs. It's important to check with your pediatrician and get his approval before your embark on any sort of supplementation program.

Now, with these general principles in mind, it's time to move on to specific diets for your child from age one to five. You'll notice that the diets are divided into four main sections, according to the age of your youngster and the calories he needs each day.

Chapter eight contains the Brain Food menus for children from the first to the second birthday. Chapter nine includes foods for youngsters from the second to the third birthday. Chapter ten is devoted to the Brain Food program for children from the third birthday to the fourth birthday. And chapter eleven contains the Brain Food Diet from the fourth birthday to the sixth birthday.

Each day's menu is divided into five meals—in part because I've found that the appetites of many young children aren't suited to the three-meal schedule followed by most adults. Young stomachs are smaller, and young appetites make demands more often and are satisfied more quickly than those of adults. Perhaps most important of all, studies have demonstrated that nutrients are best utilized in small amounts in the body, rather than in large, infrequent servings.

On the other hand, nothing about this daily five-meal program is written in stone. If you find that your child responds better to a four-meal plan, or even to three meals a day, then by all means combine the foods listed on any given day into fewer than five sittings. By the same token, if you find that your son or daughter operates better with six meals than five, then spread the foods out more.

A word of caution: Don't abandon the five-meal plan just because it's inconvenient for you as a parent, or because you tend to allow your child to snack on sweets or other junk foods that spoil his appetite for five good meals.

I recognize the fact that any given day's menu may not contain foods that are convenient or palatable for you to prepare for your child. To make the substitution of other foods easier for you, we've included the number of calories contained in each serving as a numerical figure in parentheses.

Also, the food group each serving represents—protein, fat, or carbohydrate—is indicated in the second set of parentheses as *p, f,* or *c.* Some foods have significant amounts of nutrients from two or even three of these food groups, and these multinutrient items are indicated by the appropriate extra letters.

Caution: If you decide to substitute one dish for another, be sure that both the calorie amounts *and* the protein, fat, and carbohydrate contents are comparable.

The main idea in this program is to *get the best brain food possible into your child.* We'll discuss food strategies in more detail in the last chapter. But for now, just remember that your main task is to present the child's food in an attractive and manageable way so that you maximize brain growth. The foods in these diets have been organized by expert dieticians in accordance with general principles of dietary balance so your child will experience the best overall development possible. .Also, the foods have been chosen so that they conform to the Mother's Milk Principle and the other fundamentals of *The Brain Food Diet for Children.*

Now, let's consider the fifteen-day diet plan for a youngster between his first and second birthday.

8

The Brain Food Diet for Children, Ages One to Two

The following fifteen days of menus for children, from the first to the second birthday, are based on the principles outlined in the previous chapter. The approximate daily number of calories is 1100, though there is some variation from day to day.

Remember that the numbers in parentheses represent the number of calories for each item. The letters *p,c,f* refer, respectively, to whether the food is primarily protein, carbohydrate or fat—or a combination of two or more of these food groups. If you want to substitute one item for another mentioned among the sample foods, be sure that *both* (1) the calorie and (2) the protein-carbohydrate-fat values are the same. Otherwise, the brain food balance of the diet may be upset, and the over-all nutritional and caloric balance may be undermined as well.

Finally, if you do choose to substitute one item for another, you can often achieve equivalency by simple division or multiplication of the calorie values: That is, if one item is "(70) *(p,c,f)*" and a second is "(140) *(p,c,f)*," just divide the second by two to get "(70) *(p,c,f)*," or the exact equivalent of the first.

DAY 1

Meal 1:

    ½ cup tomato juice (**24**) *(c)*
    ½ waffle (**35**) *(c)*, with
    1 teaspoon margarine (**35**) *(f)*
    ½ cup whole milk (**75**) *(p,c,f)*

Meal 2:

    ½ cup lentil soup (**130**) *(p,c,f)*
    1 oz. natural cheese cubes (**107**) *(p,f)*, over ½ slice rye
        bread (**28**) *(c)*
    ½ cup whole milk (**75**) *(p,c,f)*

Meal 3:

    1 oz. broiled veal chop (**66**) *(p,f)*
    2 teaspoons margarine (**70**) *(f)*
    ½ cup cooked zucchini (**11**) *(c)*
    ½ cup soft ice cream (**164**) *(p,c,f)*
    ¼ cup apple juice (**30**) *(c)*

Meal 4:

    ½ banana (**42**) *(c)*
    5 strawberries (**18**) *(c)*
    ½ cup whole milk (**75**) *(p,c,f)*

Meal 5:

    2 small peanut butter cookies (**84**) *(p,c,f)*
    ½ cup fruit juice (**64**) *(c)*

DAY 2

Meal 1:

¼ sliced apple, 2 orange sections, ¼ banana (58) (c)
½ toasted pumpernickel bagel (70) (c)
1 tablespoon cream cheese (49) (p,f)
½ cup whole milk (75) (p,c,f)

Meal 2:

½ cup fish chowder (100) (p,c,f)
4–5 whole wheat crackers (72) (c)
½ cup apple juice (60) (c)
½ oz. cheese (53) (p,f)

Meal 3:

½ cup yogurt (75) (p,c,f)
¼ cup berries (21) (c)
2 Graham crackers (54) (c)

Meal 4:

1 oz. broiled chicken (35) (p)
2 tablespoons mashed potatoes (22) (c)
2 teaspoons margarine (70) (f)
½ cup steamed zucchini sticks (11) (c)
½ cup juice (64) (c)
½ cup whole milk (75) (p,c,f)

Meal 5:

½ cup plain ice cream (139) (p,c,f), with 1 tablespoon hot fruit topping (15) (c)

HOT FRUIT SAUCE:

RECIPE: Place in saucepot 1 chopped apple, 1 chopped pear, ½ cup berries, ½ cup unsweetened pineapples, and ½ cup unsweetened pineapple juice. Cook until mixture thickens, adding a pinch of cornstarch if desired. Cool slightly before pouring over ice cream.

1 small peanut butter cookie (42) (p,c,f)

DAY 3

Meal 1:

  ¼ cup pineapple chunks (**17**) (*c*)
  1 egg, scrambled (**78**) (*p,f*)
  ½ corn muffin (**65**) (*c*)
  1 teaspoon margarine (**35**) (*f*)
  ½ cup whole milk (**75**) (*p,c,f*)

Meal 2:

  1 peanut butter cookie (**42**) (*p,c,f*)
  ½ cup yogurt (**75**) (*p,c,f*)

Meal 3:

  ½ cup green pea soup (**35**) (*p,c*)
  1 oz. ground salmon (**30**) (*p,c,f*)
  ¼ cup creamed spinach (**30**) (*p,c,f*)
  ½ cup boiled chopped mushrooms (**10**) (*c*)
  2 teaspoons margarine (**70**) (*f*)
  ¼ cup soft ice cream (**82**) (*p,c,f*)
  ½ cup whole milk (**75**) (*p,c,f*)

Meal 4:

  ½ oz. ground chicken (**176**) (*p*)
  1 tablespoon mashed boiled potatoes (**11**) (*c*)
  ¼ cup boiled ground carrots (**11**) (*c*)
  ¼ cup boiled ground green beans (**10**) (*c*), fried in 2
    teaspoons margarine (**70**) (*f*)
  ½ cup whole milk (**75**) (*p,c,f*)

Meal 5:

  ⅓ cup cottage cheese (**68**) (*p,c,f*)
  5 whole grain crackers (**48**) (*c*)
  ½ cup juice (**64**) (*c*)

DAY 4

Meal 1:

⅓ cup warm apple cider **(40)** *(c)*

1 slice french toast **(119)** *(p,c,f)*, with ½ tablespoon peanut butter **(42)** *(p,c,f)*, blended with 1 tablespoon applesauce **(5)** *(c)* as a topping

Meal 2:

½ cup tomato soup **(40)** *(c)*

½ slice enriched whole wheat bread **(28)** *(c)*

1 teaspoon margarine **(35)** *(f)*

½ cup fruit juice **(64)** *(c)*

¼ cup ice cream **(69)** *(p,c,f)*

Meal 3:

1 oz. cheese **(103)** *(p,f)*

1 bread stick **(30)** *(c)*

½ cup cranberry juice **(81)** *(c)*

Meal 4:

1 oz. broiled ground steak **(74)** *(p,f)*

½ cup steamed cabbage **(16)** *(c)*

2 teaspoons margarine **(70)** *(f)*

½ cup whole milk **(75)** *(p,c,f)*

¼ cup watermelon **(13)** *(c)*

Meal 5:

½ cup whole milk **(75)** *(p,c,f)*

⅓ cup bran cereal **(50)** *(c)*, with ¼ cup fresh fruit **(20)** *(c)*

DAY 5

Meal 1:

½ medium unsweetened baked or steamed apple (**20**) *(c)*

1 open-face toasted cheese sandwich (**150**) *(p,c,f)*

½ cup whole milk (**75**) *(p,c,f)*

Meal 2:

½ slice banana bread (**67**) *(c)*, with 1 tablespoon cream cheese (**49**) *(p,f)*

Meal 3:

½ slice whole wheat bread (**28**) *(c)*

1 oz. ground turkey (**54**) *(p)*

2 teaspoons mayonnaise (**67**) *(f)*

¼ cup milk shake (**35**) *(p,c,f)*

1 fresh peach (**38**) *(c)*

Meal 4:

1 oz. baked fish in cheese (**77**) *(p,c,f)*

½ cup steamed ground broccoli (**29**) *(c)*

¼ cup summer squash (**7**) *(c)*

2 teaspoons margarine (**70**) *(f)*

½ cup whole milk (**75**) *(p,c,f)*

Meal 5:

1 cup whole milk (**150**) *(p,c,f)*

1 Graham cracker (**27**) *(c)*

DAY 6

Meal 1:

  ½ cup grapefruit juice (**48**) *(c)*
  1 baked egg (**82**) *(p,f)*
  ½ slice rye toast (**28**) *(c)*
  ½ teaspoon margarine (**35**) *(f)*
  ½ cup cocoa (**109**) *(p,c,f)*

Meal 2:

  ½ slice bran bread (**37**) *(c)*
  1 tablespoon peanut butter (**86**) *(f)*
  ½ cup fruit juice (**64**) *(c)*

Meal 3:

  ¼ cup orange and grapefruit sections (**41**) *(c)*, sprinkled
    with 1 tablespoon powered coconut and nuts (**60**) *(f)*
  1 cup whole milk (**150**) *(p,c,f)*

Meal 4:

  SEAFOOD SPECIAL:
  RECIPE: Take 1 oz. mixed seafood (sole, whitefish, striped bass)
  (**62**) *(p)* and broil in 3 teaspoons margarine (**105**) *(f)*. Add to ¼
  cup cooked tomato with onion, celery, and spinach (**15**) *(c)* and
  serve over ¼ cup boiled brown rice (**44**) *(c)*.
  ½ cup whole milk (**75**) *(p,c,f)*

Meal 5:

  ½ cup ice cream (**75**) *(p,c,f)*, with 2 tablespoons hot fruit
    sauce (**30**) *(c)* (see page 92)

DAY 7

Meal 1:

⅓ small banana **(28)** *(c)*
Corn meal pancake **(68)** *(c)*
1 teaspoon margarine **(35)** *(f)*
1 teaspoon honey **(20)** *(c)*
½ cup whole milk **(75)** *(p,c,f)*

Meal 2:

¼ cup avocado pear, puréed **(63)** *(c,f)*, spread on 3 whole
    wheat crackers **(48)** *(c)*
½ cup whole milk **(75)** *(p,c,f)*

Meal 3:

1 oz. broiled veal chop **(66)** *(p)*
2 small cooked carrots **(40)** *(c)*
2 teaspoons margarine **(70)** *(f)*
⅓ cup frozen juice (grape or cranberry) **(55)** *(c)*
½ cup cooked zucchini **(11)** *(c)*

Meal 4:

½ cup lentil soup **(130)** *(p,c,f)*
½ cup medium cucumber sticks, raw, peeled and sliced
    (14) *(c)*
½ slice whole wheat bread **(28)** *(c)*
1 cup whole milk **(150)** *(p,c,f)*

Meal 5:

½ cup yogurt **(75)** *(p,c,f)*, with ½ peach, mashed **(19)** *(c)*

DAY 8

Meal 1:

¼ cup grapefruit sections **(15)** *(c)*
1 deviled egg **(145)** *(p,f)*
1 teaspoon margarine **(35)** *(f)*
½ slice whole wheat bread **(28)** *(c)*
½ cup whole milk **(75)** *(p,c,f)*

Meal 2:

1 oz. natural cheese **(107)** *(p,f)*, melted on ½ slice
    pumpernickel bread **(28)** *(c)*
¼ cup unsweetened apple sauce **(20)** *(c)*
½ cup whole milk **(75)** *(p,c,f)*

Meal 3:

½ cup whole milk **(75)** *(p,c,f)*
1 raisin bran cookie **(75)** *(c,f)*

Meal 4:

½ cup ice cream with 2 tablespoons granola topping **(150)**
    (p,c,f)
½ cup juice **(64)** *(c)*

Meal 5:

1 oz. broiled ground steak **(74)** *(p,f)*
½ cup steamed spinach, finely chopped **(21)** *(c)*
1 teaspoon margarine **(35)** *(f)*
¼ cup fresh melon **(13)** *(c)*

DAY 9

Meal 1:

Small bunch of seedless grapes **(51)** *(c)*, or ¼ cup grape
juice **(41)** *(c)*

½ slice oatmeal bread **(30)** *(c)*

1 teaspoon margarine **(35)** *(f)*

½ cup whole milk **(75)** *(p,c,f)*

Meal 2:

½ cup whole milk **(75)** *(p,c,f)*

½ oz. hard natural cheese **(56)** *(p,f)*

5 small whole grain crackers **(48)** *(c)*

1 small apple peeled and coarsely grated **(44)** *(c)*

Meal 3:

1 oz. broiled chicken **(35)** *(p)*

¼ cup mashed boiled potatoes **(45)** *(c)*

½ cup boiled green beans **(20)** *(c)*, covered with

2 teaspoons margarine **(70)** *(f)*

½ cup whole milk **(75)** *(p,c,f)*

Meal 4:

1 peanut butter cookie **(84)** *(p,c,f)*

½ cup whole milk **(75)** *(p,c,f)*

Meal 5:

1 oz. broiled ground beef **(93)** *(p,f)*

1 small piece of corn bread **(105)** *(c)*

1 teaspoon margarine **(35)** *(f)*

½ cup whole milk **(75)** *(p,c,f)*

Fruit kabob **(40)** *(c)*: 5 small pieces of mixed fruit on a
stick

DAY 10

Meal 1:

¼ apple finely sliced **(22)** *(c)*

Lighthouse egg **(130)** *(p,c,f)*: 1 slice rice bread with hole cut in the middle where egg is fried

2 teaspoons margarine **(70)** *(f)* for frying

1 cup whole milk **(150)** *(p,c,f)*

Meal 2:

½ cup cottage cheese **(101)** *(p,f,c)*

2 whole grain rye wafers or crackers **(132)** *(c)*

1 slice tomato **(2.5)** *(c)*

½ cup grapefruit sections **(30)** *(c)*

Meal 3:

½ cup whole milk **(75)** *(p,c,f)*

1 raisin cookie **(75)** *(c,f)*

¼ cup sliced avocado pear **(63)** *(p,f)*

½ teaspoon mayonnaise **(17)** *(f)* garnished with paprika

Meal 4:

½ slice whole wheat bread **(28)** *(c)*

1 oz. ground turkey **(54)** *(p)*

2 teaspoons mayonnaise **(67)** *(f)*

¼ cup whole milk **(37)** *(p,c,f)*

1 fresh peach **(38)** *(c)*

Meal 5:

⅓ cup of yogurt **(50)** *(p,c,f)* with ¼ cup pineapple in small pieces **(17)** *(c)*

DAY 11

Meal 1:

½ cup apple juice (**60**) (*c*)

¼ cup hot oatmeal (**37**) (*c*). Use some apple juice instead of water to cook cereal. A few apple pieces may be added also.

1 teaspoon margarine (**35**) (*f*)

1 egg (**78**) (*p,f*) fried using 1 teaspoon margarine (**35**) (*f*)

½ cup whole milk (**75**) (*p,c,f*)

Meal 2:

1 oz. broiled mackerel (**54**) (*p,f*) flaked, in 1 teaspoon sweet oil (**35**) (*f*)

2 tablespoons mashed potatoes (**22**) (*c*)

2 teaspoons margarine (**70**) (*f*) over ¼ cup boiled green beans (**10**) (*c*)

¼ cup boiled carrots (**11**) (*c*)

½ cup juice (**64**) (*c*)

Meal 3:

HAWAIIAN TOAST:

RECIPE: On ½ English muffin place ½ oz. of ham and 1 pineapple ring, then top with 1 oz. of grated cheese. Bake or broil 15 minutes. (**230**) (*p,c,f*)

½ cup whole milk (**75**) (*p,c,f*)

Meal 4:

½ slice soft raisin bread (**30**) (*c*)

1 tablespoon peanut butter (**86**) (*p,c,f*)

½ cup orange pulp (**40**) (*c*)

Meal 5:

½ cup whole milk (**75**) (*p,c,f*)

½ banana bran muffin (**60**) (*c*)

1 teaspoon margarine (**35**) (*f*)

DAY 12

Meal 1:

   ¼ cup orange and grapefruit sections **(41)** *(c)* sprinkled
      with 1 tablespoon powdered coconut and nuts **(60)** *(f)*
   ½ cup whole milk **(75)** *(p,c,f)*

Meal 2:

   ½ whole wheat English muffin **(73)** *(c)* spread with 1
      tablespoon peanut butter **(86)** *(p,c,f)*
   ½ cup fruit juice **(30)** *(c)*

Meal 3:

   SEAFOOD SPECIAL:

   RECIPE: Broil 1 oz. of mixed seafood (flounder, sole, red snap-
   per) **(62)** *(p)* in 3 teaspoons margarine **(105)** *(f)* and place in the
   center of ¼ cup boiled brown rice **(40)** *(c)* and surround with ¼
   cup cooked tomato, celery, and spinach **(20)** *(c)*
   ½ cup whole milk **(75)** *(p,c,f)*

Meal 4:

   ½ blueberry muffin **(56)** *(c)*
   1 teaspoon margarine **(35)** *(f)*
   1 scrambled egg **(78)** *(p,f)*
   ½ cup whole milk **(75)** *(p,c,f)*

Meal 5:

   ½ cup whole yogurt **(75)** *(p,c,f)* with ¼ cup berries
      (mashed) **(20)** *(c)*

DAY 13

Meal 1:

   ½ medium peach, puréed (19) (c)
   1½ teaspoon peanut butter (42) (p,c,f,) on ½ slice raisin
        bread (30) (c)
   1 teaspoon margarine (35) (f)
   ½ cup whole milk (75) (p,c,f)

Meal 2:

   1 oatmeal cookie (80) (c,f)
   ½ cup whole milk (75) (p,c,f)

Meal 3:

   ⅓ cup macaroni and cheese (170) (p,c,f)
   ⅓ cup carrot and celery sticks (20) (c)
   1 tangerine (40) (c)
   ½ cup whole milk (75) (p,c,f)

Meal 4:

   RAINBOW SALAD:

   RECIPE: Mix ½ cup watermelon and cantaloupe balls (27) (c),
   with 1½ teaspoons chopped raisins (10) (c), then stir in 3 small
   powdered walnuts (16) (p,c,f). Pour ½ teaspoon lemon juice
   over mixture before serving.

   ½ cup whole milk (75) (p,c,f)

Meal 5:

   ½ cup black pea soup (92) (p,c)
   1 tablespoon peanut butter (86) (p,c,f) on ½ slice whole
        wheat bread (28) (c)
   ½ cup orange juice (56) (c)

DAY 14

Meal 1:
- 1 egg, scrambled **(78)** *(p,f)*
- ½ slice whole wheat bread, toasted **(28)** *(c)*
- 1 teaspoon margarine **(35)** *(f)*
- ½ cup whole milk **(75)** *(p,c,f)*

Meal 2:
- ½ cup fresh orange juice **(56)** *(c)*
- 1 tablespoon cream cheese **(49)** *(p,f)* on ½ slice cracked wheat bread **(30)** *(c)*

Meal 3:
- 2 oz. boneless ground beef **(186)** *(p,f)*
- 1 teaspoon margarine **(35)** *(f)*
- ½ cup cauliflower **(12)** *(p,c)*
- ½ cup strawberries **(28)** *(c)*
- 1 tablespoon whipped cream **(28)** *(f)*
- ½ cup whole milk **(75)** *(p,c,f)*

Meal 4:
- 2 oz. mackerel **(108)** *(p,f)*
- ½ cup spinach **(21)** *(c)*
- 1 teaspoon margarine **(35)** *(f)*
- 2 tablespoons mashed potatoes **(22)** *(c)*
- ½ cup mushrooms **(10)** *(c)*
- ½ cup whole milk **(75)** *(p,c,f)*
- 1 small plum **(22)** *(c)*

Meal 5:
- 1 cup whole milk **(150)** *(p,c,f)*
- 1 biscuit **(130)** *(c,f)*

DAY 15

Meal 1:
> ½ cup tomato juice **(24)** *(c)*
> ½ waffle **(35)** *(c)*, with 1 teaspoon margarine **(35)** *(f)*
> ½ cup whole milk **(75)** *(p,c,f)*

Meal 2:
> ½ cup lentil soup **(130)** *(p,c,f)*
> 1 oz. natural cheese cubes **(107)** *(p,c,f)*, over ½ slice rye
>   bread **(28)** *(c)*
> ½ cup whole milk **(75)** *(p,c,f)*

Meal 3:
> 1 oz. broiled veal chop **(66)** *(p,f)*
> 2 teaspoons margarine **(70)** *(f)*
> ½ cup cooked zucchini **(11)** *(c)*
> ½ cup soft ice cream **(164)** *(p,c,f)*
> ¼ cup apple juice **(40)** *(c)*

Meal 4:
> ½ banana **(42)** *(c)*
> 5 strawberries **(18)** *(c)*
> ½ cup whole milk **(75)** *(p,c,f)*

Meal 5:
> 2 small peanut butter cookies **(84)** *(p,c,f)*
> ½ cup fruit juice **(64)** *(c)*

9

The Brain Food Diet for Children, Ages Two to Three

The fifteen days of menus in this chapter are intended for children between the second and third birthdays. The foods suggested each day are balanced according to the principles outlined in chapter seven, with approximately 1300 calories provided daily. Also, remember that the numbers in parentheses represent the calorie values of each item. Finally, the letters *p,c,f* in parentheses indicate, respectively, whether the item is primarily protein, carbohydrate, or fat—or a combination of these food groups.

DAY 1

Meal 1:

½ cup unsweetened applesauce (41) *(c)*
Corn meal pancake (68) *(c)*
1 teaspoon margarine (35) *(f)*
6 oz. whole milk (112) *(p,c,f)*

Meal 2:

½ cup juice (64) *(c)*
½ oz. natural cheese (53) *(p,c,f)* melted on 1 soya muffin
   (119) *(c)*
½ cup salad of tomato, avocado, mushroom, and lettuce
   (50) *(c,f)*, and 2 teaspoons oil (70) *(f)* as a dressing

Meal 3:

MINIATURE PIZZA:
RECIPE: Take ½ English muffin (69) *(c)* and spread with 1 tablespoon tomato sauce (7) *(c)*. Top with 1 slice mozzarella
cheese (94) *(p,f)* and sprinkle on ¼ cup green pepper slices (4)
(c). Toast in oven for 15 minutes.
   1 cup whole milk (150) *(p,c,f)*

Meal 4:

½ cup fish chowder (100) *(p,c,f)*
2–3 whole wheat crackers (40) *(c)*
½ cup cole slaw (86) *(c,f)*
½ cup cranberry juice (81) *(c)*

Meal 5:

½ cup berries (43) *(c)*
½ cup yogurt (75) *(p,c,f)*
1 oatmeal cookie (80) *(c)*

DAY 2

Meal 1:

½ cup warm apple cider **(60)** *(c)*

1 waffle **(70)** *(c)* spread with 1 tablespoon peanut butter **(86)** *(p,c,f)* mixed with 2 teaspoons applesauce **(3)** *(c)*

½ cup whole milk **(75)** *(p,c,f)*

Meal 2:

½ cup lentil soup **(130)** *(p,c,f)*

1 hard boiled egg **(78)** *(p,f)*

3–4 Rye wafers **(72)** *(c)*

½ cup fruit **(41)** *(c)*

½ cup whole milk **(75)** *(p,c,f)*

Meal 3:

1½ oz. broiled veal chop **(99)** *(p,f)*

3 tablespoons mashed potatoes **(33)** *(c)*

1 teaspoon margarine **(35)** *(f)*

½ cup steamed cauliflower **(12)** *(p,c)*

½ cup whole milk **(75)** *(p,c,f)*

Meal 4:

1 slice raisin whole wheat bread **(60)** *(c)* spread with 1 tablespoon peanut butter **(86)** *(p,c,f)*

½ cup apple juice **(60)** *(c)*

⅓ cup vanilla pudding **(110)** *(c)*

Meal 5:

Fruit kabob **(40)** *(c)*: 5 small pieces of mixed fruit on a stick

1 cup whole milk **(150)** *(p,c,f)*

DAY 3

Meal 1:
   ½ cup pineapple chunks **(32)** *(c)*
   1 corn muffin **(130)** *(c)*
   1 teaspoon margarine **(35)** *(f)*
   ½ cup whole milk **(75)** *(p,c,f)*
   1 hard boiled egg **(78)** *(p,f)*

Meal 2:
   1½ oz. roast lamb **(103)** *(p,f)*
   ⅓ cup brussels sprouts **(20)** *(c)*
   ¼ cup grapefruit and mandarin orange sections **(46)** *(c)*,
      covered with 1 tablespoon ground nuts and coconut
      (60) *(f,c)*
   ½ cup whole milk **(75)** *(p,c,f)*

Meal 3:
   ½ cup whole milk **(75)** *(p,c,f)*
   Fruit kabob **(40)** *(c)*: 5 small pieces of mixed fruit on a
      stick

Meal 4:

   HUMMUS:
RECIPE: Soak, and then cook for approximately 1½ hours, ½
cup dried chickpeas (garbanzo beans). To the drained and
mashed beans blend in one small clove of garlic finely
chopped, 1 teaspoon chopped onion, ⅛ cup of Tahini, 1 dash of
Tamiri, and 1 teaspoon finely chopped parsley **(70)** *(p,c)*.
   ½ small size Syrian pocket bread **(48)** *(c)*
   3 tablespoons dried fruit—figs, raisins, prunes **(60)** *(c)*
   6 oz. whole milk **(112)** *(p,c,f)*

Meal 5:
   1 cup whole milk **(150)** *(p,c,f)*
   1 raisin cookie **(75)** *(c,f)*
   1 peanut butter cookie **(84)** *(p,c,f)*

DAY 4

Meal 1:

½ apple cut in wedges **(44)** *(c)*

½ toasted pumpernickel bagel **(70)** *(c)* spread with 1
tablespoon cream cheese **(49)** *(p,f)*

4 oz. cocoa **(109)** *(p,c,f)*

Meal 2:

1 slice raisin bread **(60)** *(c)* spread with 1 tablespoon
peanut butter **(86)** *(p,c,f)*

½ cup apple juice **(60)** *(c)*

Meal 3:

YOK YOUNG STIR-FRIED DINNER:

RECIPE: Use 3 teaspoons oil **(105)** *(f)* in a wok or deep frying
pan to stir and fry ½ cup of the following mixed vegetables:
chopped broccoli, carrots, mushrooms, onions, snow peas, celery, bamboo shoots, and water chestnuts **(45)** *(c)*. To this mixture add 1½ oz. browned ground beef **(139)** *(p,f)* and 1 teaspoon
powdered almonds **(30)** *(p,c,f)*, serve over ¼ cup brown rice **(44)**
(c) and season with 2 teaspoons soy sauce.

½ cup orange sections **(47)** *(c)*

½ cup whole milk **(75)** *(p,c,f)*

Meal 4:

½ cup fruit salad: strawberries, banana, avocado,
pineapple **(41)** *(c,f)*, over ½ cup yogurt **(75)** *(p,c,f)*

Meal 5:

TOMATO VOLCANO:

RECIPE: Scoop out the center of 1 tomato **(33)** *(c)* and fill with a
mixture of ¼ cup tuna in oil **(192)** *(p,f)*, 1 teaspoon margarine
(35) *(f)*, and ¼ cup finely chopped cucumbers, celery, onion,
parsley, green pepper, and tomato contents **(20)** *(c)*. Steam the
tomato and its contents for 10 to 15 minutes.

1 cup whole milk **(150)** *(p,c,f)*

DAY 5

Meal 1:
   ½ cup cranberry juice **(81)** *(c)*
   1 slice whole wheat toast **(28)** *(c)* spread with **1**
      tablespoon peanut butter **(86)** *(p,c,f)*
   1 cup whole milk **(150)** *(p,c,f)*

Meal 2:
   ½ cup vegetable beef soup **(67)** *(p,c)*
   5–6 whole wheat crackers **(50)** *(c)*
   1 tangerine **(40)** *(c)*
   6 oz. whole milk **(112)** *(p,c,f)*

Meal 3:
   ½ cup Waldorf salad **(70)** *(f,c)*, containing apple slices,
      celery pieces, small nuts, and mayonnaise
   ½ cup whole milk **(75)** *(p,c,f)*

Meal 4:
   1 oz. boneless ground beef **(93)** *(p,f)*
   ¼ cup mashed potatoes **(45)** *(c)*
   ½ cup tossed avocado, tomato, cucumber salad **(70)** *(p,c,f)*
      with 1 teaspoon vinegar and oil dressing `(77)` *(f)*
   ½ cup whole milk **(75)** *(p,c,f)*

Meal 5:
   1 cup whole milk **(150)** *(p,c,f)*
   1 peanut butter cookie **(84)** *(p,c,f)* crumbled over ½ cup
      ice cream **(139)** *(p,c,f)*

DAY 6

Meal 1:

    ½ cup tomato juice **(24)** *(c)*
    1 poached egg **(78)** *(p,f)*
    ½ whole wheat English muffin **(73)** *(c)*
    1 teaspoon margarine **(35)** *(f)*
    6 oz. whole milk **(112)** *(p,c,f)*

Meal 2:

POCKET TURKEY SANDWICH:

RECIPE: Take ½ medium size Syrian pocket bread **(68)** *(c)* and stuff it with a mixture of 1 oz. cooked turkey **(54)** *(p)*, 2 teaspoons mayonnaise **(67)** *(f)* and ¼ cup chopped lettuce and tomato **(10)** *(c)*.

    Fresh plum **(22)** *(c)*
    6 oz. whole milk **(112)** *(p,c,f)*

Meal 3:

    1½ oz. cheese sticks **(170)** *(p,f)*
    ½ cup apricot juice **(61)** *(c)*

Meal 4:

    2 oz. broiled sole **(110)** *(p)* with lemon
    ¼ cup sweet corn **(41)** *(c)*
    2 teaspoons margarine **(70)** *(f)*
    ½ cup whole milk **(75)** *(p,c,f)*

Meal 5:

    ½ cup yogurt **(75)** *(p,c,f)*
    ¼ cup berries **(21)** *(c)*

DAY 7

Meal 1:
> ½ cup grapefruit sections (**30**) *(c)*
> Lighthouse egg (**130**) *(p,c,f)*: 1 slice oatmeal bread, with
>   hole cut out for 1 egg and fried in 2 teaspoons
>   margarine
> ½ cup whole milk (**75**) *(p,c,f)*

Meal 2:
> ½ whole wheat English muffin (**73**) *(c)*
> 1 tablespoon peanut butter (**86**) *(p,c,f)*
> ½ cup whole milk (**75**) *(p,c,f)*

Meal 3:

SEAFOOD SUPREME:
RECIPE: Flake ¼ cup tuna fish (**96**) *(p,f)* on 1 slice oatmeal bread
(**60**) *(c)*, sprinkle 1 oz. shredded Swiss cheese (**100**) *(p,f)* on top
and melt in oven.
> ½ cup pineapple chunks (**32**) *(c)*
> 6 oz. whole milk (**112**) *(p,c,f)*

Meal 4:
> ½ cup ice cream (**139**) *(p,c,f)* topped with 2 tablespoons
>   granola (**20**) *(c)*
> ½ cup apple juice (**64**) *(c)*

Meal 5:
> 1½ oz. baked ham (**105**) *(p,f)*
> ½ sweet potato (**70**) *(c)*
> ⅓ cup applesauce (**27**) *(c)*
> 6 oz. whole milk (**112**) *(p,c,f)*

DAY 8

Meal 1:

    ½ cup orange juice (**60**) (*c*)
    ½ cup hot oatmeal (**74**) (*c*)
    1 teaspoon margarine (**35**) (*f*)
    6 oz. whole milk (**112**) (*p,c,f*)

Meal 2:

    1½ oz. roasted chicken (**52**) (*p*)
    ¼ cup wild rice (**54**) (*c*)
    ¼ cup boiled waxed beans (**10**) (*c*)
    2 teaspoons margarine (**70**) (*f*)
    ½ small apple in wedges (**26**) (*c*)
    ½ cup whole milk (**75**) (*p,c,f*)

Meal 3:

HAND-MEAT PIE:
RECIPE: Take 1½ oz. broiled ground beef (**139**) (*p,f*) and form into
a thick patty. Wrap 1 oz. pastry (**150**) (*c,f*) around the meat. Seal
loose edges with a fork and puncture each side once with a
fork. Bake for 30 minutes or until golden brown.

    ½ cup cooked yellow squash (**14**) (*c*)
    ½ cup whole milk (**75**) (*p,c,f*)

Meal 4:

    ½ cup Sight Savers Salad: ½ cup grated carrots (**22**) (*c*), 2
        tablespoons raisins (**58**) (*c*), 1 tablespoon mayonnaise
        (**101**) (*f*), and 2 slices avocado pear (**47**) (*f,c*).
    ½ cup whole milk (**75**) (*p,c,f*)

Meal 5:

CELERY BARGE:
RECIPE: 1 stick celery spread over with a mixture of ½ oz.
Cheddar cheese and 2 teaspoons mayonnaise (**67**) (*p,f*).
    ½ cup whole milk (**75**) (*p,c,f*)

DAY 9

Meal 1:

   ½ cup grapefruit and orange wedges **(38)** *(c)*
   1 egg **(78)** *(p,c,f)* fried with 1 teaspoon margarine **(35)** *(f)*
   1 slice whole wheat toast **(56)** *(c)*
   6 oz. whole milk **(112)** *(p,c,f)*

Meal 2:

   1 cup whole milk **(150)** *(p,c,f)*
   1 peanut butter cookie **(84)** *(p,c,f)*

Meal 3:

   1½ oz. boneless ground beef **(139)** *(p,f)*
   2 tablespoons mashed potatoes **(22)** *(c)* topped with 1½
      teaspoons margarine **(52)** *(f)*
   ⅓ cup boiled green beans **(15)** *(c)*
   6 oz. whole milk **(112)** *(p,c,f)*

Meal 4:

   TUNA TANTALIZER:

RECIPE: Take ⅓ cup macaroni with cheese sauce **(170)** *(p,c,f)*
and mix with ¼ cup oil-packed tuna **(96)** *(p,f)*. Put mixture in
dish and top with 2 tablespoons bread crumbs **(25)** *(c)*. Bake in
oven at 350 for 25 minutes or until golden brown.
   1 peach **(38)** *(c)*
   6 oz. whole milk **(112)** *(p,c,f)*

Meal 5:

   ½ cup whole milk **(75)** *(p,c,f)*
   ½ cup cottage cheese **(101)** *(p,c,f)*
   Fruit kabob **(40)** *(c)*: 5 small pieces of mixed fruit on a
      stick

DAY 10

Meal 1:

    ½ cup cottage cheese (101) (p,c,f)
    ½ whole wheat English muffin (73) (c)
    2 teaspoons margarine (70) (f)
    ½ cup apple juice (60) (c)

Meal 2:

    1½ oz. broiled sole (80) (p) with ½ oz. natural cheese (55) (p,c,f)
    ¼ cup sweet corn (41) (c)
    2 teaspoons margarine (70) (f)
    1 nectarine (32) (c)
    6 oz. whole milk (112) (p,c,f)

Meal 3:

    1 cup whole milk (150) (p,c,f)
    ½ small banana on a stick (42) (c)

Meal 4:

TURKEY SANDWICH:
RECIPE: Make sandwich with 1 slice whole wheat bread (56) (c), 1 oz. boiled ground turkey (54) (p), and 1 tablespoon mayonnaise (101) (f). Sprinkle with chopped lettuce and tomato (5) (c).
    ½ cup raw zucchini sticks (11) (c)
    6 oz. whole milk (112) (p,c,f)

Meal 5:

    1 slice cinnamon raisin bread (60) (c) spread with 2 teaspoons peanut butter (56) (p,c,f)
    6 oz. whole milk (112) (p,c,f)

DAY 11

Meal 1:

> Hawaiian toast **(230)** *(p,c,f)* (see page 101)
> 6 oz. whole milk **(112)** *(p,c,f)*

Meal 2:

> 1 slice raisin whole wheat bread **(60)** *(c)* spread with 1
>   tablespoon peanut butter **(86)** *(p,c,f)*
> ½ cup whole milk **(75)** *(p,c,f)*

Meal 3:

> ½ cup lentil soup **(130)** *(p,c,f)*

  VEGI PUFFS:
RECIPE: Place ½ cup chopped broccoli and green beans with 2
tablespoons cheese sauce in 3 in. pastry shell **(110)** *(p,c,f)*. Bake
for 30 minutes in oven at 350.

> ½ cup whole milk **(75)** *(p,c,f)*

Meal 4:

> 1½ oz. broiled veal chop **(99)** *(p,f)*
> 3 tablespoons mashed potatoes **(33)** *(c)*
> 2 teaspoons margarine **(70)** *(f)*
> ⅓ cup zucchini **(11)** *(c)*
> ½ cup whole milk **(75)** *(p,c,f)*

Meal 5:

  YOGURT YUM YUM:
RECIPE: ½ cup contains the following: ½ cup yogurt **(75)** *(p,c,f)*
blended with ⅓ cup strawberries, pears, banana pieces **(55)** *(c)*
and 2 tablespoons finely ground nuts and coconut **(90)** *(p,c,f)*.

DAY 12

Meal 1:

    2 small figs **(40)** *(c)*
    Creamed corn omelet **(109)** *(p,c,f)*
    ½ slice whole wheat toast **(28)** *(c)*
    6 oz. whole milk **(112)** *(p,c,f)*

Meal 2:

    1 oz. sliced beef **(93)** *(p,f)*
    1 cup cauliflower, broccoli, green pepper, carrots, and
       celery **(31)** *(c)* stir fried in 2 teaspoons sweet oil **(70)**
       (f)
    ½ cup whole milk **(75)** *(p,c,f)*

Meal 3:

    ½ cup orange juice **(56)** *(c)*
    1 buttermilk biscuit **(82)** *(c,f)* covered with ½ oz. melted
       cheese **(53)** *(p,c,f)*
    1 cup salad of tomato, avocado, mushroom, lettuce
       (70) *(p,c,f)*, covered with 1 teaspoon oil and dash of
       vinegar **(26)** *(f)*

Meal 4:

    2 tablespoons coconut, almonds, pecans, sesame seeds,
       finely ground **(90)** *(p,c,f)* and sprinkled over ⅓ cup
       pineapple, pear, and orange pieces **(45)** *(c)*
    6 oz. whole milk **(112)** *(p,c,f)*

Meal 5:

    1½ oz. meat loaf **(69)** *(p,c,f)*
    ¼ cup finely chopped spinach **(14)** *(c)*
    ¼ cup cooked carrots **(11)** *(c)*
    2 teaspoons margarine **(70)** *(f)*
    ½ cup whole milk **(75)** *(p,c,f)*
    ½ cup melon **(26)** *(c)*

DAY 13

Meal 1:

Small bunch of seedless grapes **(51)** *(c)*
1 slice oatmeal toast **(60)** *(c)* spread with 1 tablespoon
    peanut butter **(86)** *(p,c,f)*
6 oz. whole milk **(112)** *(p,c,f)*

Meal 2:

PRUNE WHIP:
RECIPE: Take ¼ cup milk **(37)** *(p,c,f)* and mix with ½ cup plain
yogurt **(75)** *(p,c,f)*. Blend mixture with 2 water soaked and
drained prunes **(60)** *(c)* until thick in the blender.
2 Graham crackers **(54)** *(c)*

Meal 3:

½ cup macaroni and cheese **(170)** *(p,c,f)*
¼ cup carrot and celery sticks **(10)** *(c)*
6 oz. whole milk **(112)** *(p,c,f)*

Meal 4:

2 raisin cookies **(150)** *(c,f)*
1 cup whole milk **(150)** *(p,c,f)*

Meal 5:

1½ oz. roast pork **(139)** *(p,f)*
⅓ cup hash brown potatoes **(157)** *(p,c,f)*
⅓ cup steamed summer squash **(19)** *(c)*
6 oz. whole milk **(112)** *(p,c,f)*

DAY 14

Meal 1:

½ cup orange juice (**56**) (*c*)
½ banana bran muffin (**60**) (*c*)
1 teaspoon margarine (**35**) (*f*)
½ cup whole milk (**75**) (*p,c,f*)
Hard boiled egg (**78**) (*p,c,f*)

Meal 2:

½ cup whole milk (**75**) (*p,c,f*)
⅓ cup ice cream (**92**) (*p,c,f*) with topping of ¼ sliced
   banana (**21**) (*c*)

Meal 3:

1½ oz. mixed seafood (codfish, haddock, halibut) (**111**)
   (*p,f*) cooked in 2 teaspoons margarine (**70**) (*f*)
¼ cup rice (**41**) (*c*)
½ cup tossed salad (**20**) (*c*)
1 tablespoon oil (**105**) (*f*) with dash of vinegar
½ cup whole milk (**75**) (*p,c,f*)

Meal 4:

1 oz. cheese, cubed (**110**) (*p,f*)
2 bread sticks (**60**) (*c*)
½ cup apricot juice (**61**) (*c*)

Meal 5:

1½ oz. broiled beef (**90**) (*p*)
½ cup lettuce and tomato, with 1 teaspoon mayonnaise
   (**35**) (*c,f*)
¼ cup grapefruit and mandarin orange sections (**46**) (*c*)
½ cup whole milk (**75**) (*p,c,f*)

DAY 15

Meal 1:
- ½ cup orange juice (56) (c)
- 1 soft-cooked egg (78) (p,f)
- 1 teaspoon margarine (35) (f)
- ¼ cup enriched farina (70) (c)
- ½ cup whole milk (75) (p,c,f)

Meal 2:
- 1 oz. veal cutlet (79) (p,f)
- ¼ cup bran flakes (26) (c)
- ½ cup cooked green beans (20) (c)
- ½ cup cooked cauliflower (12) (p,c)
- 1 tomato in wedges (22) (c)
- ½ cup whole milk (75) (p,c,f)

Meal 3:
- 1 oz. cooked beef (ground chuck) (93) (p,f)
- 2 tablespoons mashed potatoes (22) (c)
- 1 teaspoon margarine (35) (f)
- ½ cup fresh carrot rings (10) (c)
- ½ cup tossed salad: tomato, lettuce, cucumber (20) (c)
- 1 teaspoon mayonnaise (35) (f)
- 6 oz. whole milk (112) (p,f,c)

Meal 4:
- ¼ cup lentil soup (65) (p,c,f)

SEAFOOD SANDWICH:
RECIPE: Mix ¼ cup tuna (60) (p,f) with 2 teaspoons of mayonnaise (70) (f) and spread over 1 slice of whole wheat bread (56) (c) cut into 2 parts and serve as open-faced sandwich.
- 1 peach (38) (c)

Meal 5:
- 1 cup whole milk (150) (p,c,f)
- 2 cheese crackers (9) (p,c,f)

10

The Brain Food
Diet for Children,
Ages Three to Four

The fifteen days of menus in this chapter are intended for children between the third and fourth birthdays. As with the previous two chapters, the foods suggested each day are balanced according to the principles outlined in chapter seven—but in this case, approximately 1400 to 1500 calories are provided daily.

Also, continue to keep in mind that the numbers in parentheses represent the calorie values of each item. The letters *p,c,f* in parentheses indicate, respectively, whether the item is primarily protein, carbohydrate, or fat—or a combination of these food groups.

DAY 1

Meal 1:
   2 small apricots **(40)** *(c)*
   1 slice date nut bread **(270)** *(c)*
   1 tablespoon cream cheese **(49)** *(p,f)*
   1 cup whole milk **(150)** *(p,c,f)*

Meal 2:
   ½ slice whole wheat toast **(28)** *(c)*
   1 tablespoon peanut butter **(86)** *(p,c,f)*
   ½ cup whole milk **(75)** *(p,c,f)*

Meal 3:
   ¾ cup lentil vegetable soup **(83)** *(p,c)*
   5–6 rye crackers **(132)** *(c)*
   ½ cup fresh fruit salad **(41)** *(c)*
   6 oz. whole milk **(112)** *(p,c,f)*

Meal 4:
   Miniature pizza **(170)** *(p,c,f)* (see page 107)
   ½ cup tossed green salad **(10)** *(c)*
   1 tablespoon oil and vinegar dressing **(77)** *(f)*
   ½ cup melon **(26)** *(c)*
   6 oz. whole milk **(112)** *(p,c,f)*

Meal 5:

RICH MILK SHAKE:
RECIPE: 1 egg **(78)** *(p,c,f)*, ½ cup fruit **(40)** *(c)*, ½ cup yogurt **(75)** *(p,c,f)*, and ½ cup milk **(75)** *(p,c,f)* all mixed in blender until thick and foamy.

DAY 2

Meal 1:

 Small bunch of seedless grapes **(51)** *(c)*
Cheese Toast: 1 oz. natural cheese **(107)** *(p,c,f)*, on 1 slice
rye bread **(56)** *(c)*, toasted
 6 oz. whole milk **(112)** *(p,c,f)*

Meal 2:

 ½ cup vegetable bean soup **(55)** *(p,c)*

TOMATO VOLCANO:

RECIPE: Scoop out the center of one tomato **(20)** *(c)* and fill with
a mixture of ¼ cup tuna in oil **(96)**, *(p,f)* 1 tablespoon mayonnaise **(101)** *(f)* and 1 teaspoon of chopped broiled green pepper,
celery, onion **(8)** *(c)*.
 1 nectarine **(32)** *(c)*
 6 oz. whole milk **(112)** *(p,c,f)*

Meal 3:

 Fruit salad: ¼ cup strawberries, avocado, banana, and pineapple **(32)** *(p,c,f)*
 1 teaspoon grape nuts **(12)** *(p,c)*
 ½ cup ice cream **(139)** *(p,c,f)*

Meal 4:

YOK YOUNG STIR-FRIED DINNER:

RECIPE: Use 2 teaspoons oil **(70)** *(f)* in a wok or deep frying pan
to stir and fry ½ cup of vegetables including chopped celery,
snow peas, onions, mushrooms, broccoli, carrots, water chestnuts, and bamboo shoots **(45)** *(c)*. To this mixture add 2 oz.
browned ground beef **(186)** *(p,f)* and 1 teaspoon powdered
almonds **(30)** *(p,c,f)*. Serve over ¼ cup brown rice **(44)** *(c)* and
season with 2 teaspoons soy sauce.
 ½ cup orange juice **(56)** *(c)*

Meal 5:

 6 oz. whole milk **(112)** *(p,c,f)*
 ½ banana on a stick **(42)** *(c)*
 Peanut butter cookie **(84)** *(p,c,f)*

DAY 3

Meal 1:
   ½ cup tomato juice **(24)** *(c)*
   1 scrambled egg **(78)** *(p,f)*
   1 blueberry muffin **(112)** *(c)*
   3 teaspoons margarine **(105)** *(f)*
   6 oz. whole milk **(112)** *(p,c,f)*

Meal 2:
   ½ cup mixed fruit juice **(64)** *(c)*
   1 slice bran bread **(74)** *(c)*
   1 oz. cheese **(110)** *(p,c,f)*

Meal 3:
   2 oz. baked chicken **(70)** *(p)*
   ⅓ cup wild rice **(74)** *(c)*
   2 slices tomato **(5)** *(c)*
   6 oz. whole milk **(112)** *(p,c,f)*

Meal 4:
   1½ oz. broiled steak **(111)** *(p,f)*
   ⅓ cup mashed potatoes **(60)** *(c)*
   ⅓ cup steamed carrots **(15)** *(c)*
   2 teaspoons margarine **(70)** *(f)*
   6 oz. whole milk **(112)** *(p,c,f)*

Meal 5:
   ½ cup vanilla ice cream **(139)** *(p,c,f)*
   2 tablespoons hot fruit sauce **(30)** *(c)* (see page 92)
   1 raisin bran cookie **(75)** *(c,f)*

DAY 4

Meal 1:
    ½ cup hot apple cider (60) (c)
    Hawaiian toast (230) (p,f,c) (see page 101)

Meal 2:
    ½ cup bean soup (60) (c)
  3–4 whole wheat crackers (56) (c)
    ⅔ cup fruit juice frozen on a stick (43) (c)
    6 oz. whole milk (112) (p,c,f)

Meal 3:
    ½ cup orange juice (56) (c)
    1 egg salad (145) (p,f) in ½ medium size Syrian pocket
       bread (68) (c)
    ½ cup strawberries and bananas (40) (c)
    6 oz. whole milk (112) (p,c,f)

Meal 4:
    1½ oz. roast pork (139) (p,f)
    ⅓ cup steamed zucchini (11) (c)
    1 teaspoon margarine (35) (f)
    1 plum (22) (c)
    6 oz. whole milk (112) (p,c,f)

Meal 5:
    ½ cup grapefruit and mandarin sections (40) (c)
    1 slice avocado pear (80) (c,f) sprinkled with 2
       tablespoons grated coconut and nuts (90) (p,c,f)
    6 oz. whole milk (112) (p,c,f)

DAY 5

Meal 1:

   ½ grapefruit (41) *(c)*
   1 stuffed egg (145) *(p,f)*
   2 teaspoons margarine (70) *(f)*
   ½ cup whole milk (75) *(p,c,f)*

Meal 2:

   GRILLED CHEESE SANDWICH:
   RECIPE: Cut 1 slice whole wheat raisin bread (60) *(c)* in half.
   Place 1 oz. natural cheese (110) *(p,c,f)* between the bread
   pieces. Use 1 teaspoon margarine (35) *(f)* to grill both outer sides
   of the bread.
   ½ cup prune juice (96) *(c)*

Meal 3:

   2 oz. roasted chicken (70) *(p)*
   ¼ cup boiled wild rice (54) *(c)*
   2 teaspoons margarine (70) *(f)*
   ½ cup Sight Savers Salad (30) *(f,c)* (see page 114)
   ½ cup shredded raw carrots (25) *(c)*
   1 tablespoon raisins (29) *(c)*
   1 small plum (22) *(c)*
   6 oz. whole milk (112) *(p,c,f)*

Meal 4:

   2 oz. baked fish in cheese (154) *(p,c,f)*
   ¼ cup mashed potatoes (60) *(c)*
   2 teaspoons margarine (70) *(f)*
   ½ cup cooked yellow squash (14) *(c)*
   6 oz. whole milk (112) *(p,c,f)*

Meal 5:

   1 cup cocoa (218) *(p,c,f)*
   1 raisin bran cookie (75) *(p,c,f)*

DAY 6

Meal 1:
- ¼ cantaloupe in slices **(30)** *(c)*
- 1 oatmeal muffin **(104)** *(c)*
- 1 teaspoon margarine **(35)** *(f)*
- ½ cup whole milk **(75)** *(p,c,f)*

Meal 2:
- ½ cup orange sections **(47)** *(c)*

TURKEY POCKET SANDWICH:
RECIPE: Take ½ medium size Syrian pocket bread **(68)** *(c)* and fill with a mixture of ¼ cup chopped lettuce and tomato **(10)** *(c)*, 2 oz. turkey cut in small pieces **(108)** *(p)*, and 1 tablespoon mayonnaise **(101)** *(f)*.
- 1 cup whole milk **(150)** *(p,c,f)*

Meal 3:
- 1 oz. cheese cubes **(110)** *(p,f)*
- 2 bread sticks **(60)** *(c)*
- 10 seedless grapes **(25)** *(c)*
- ½ cup apple juice **(60)** *(c)*

Meal 4:
- 1 serving salmon loaf **(119)** *(p,c,f)*
- ¼ cup sweet corn **(41)** *(c)*
- 1 teaspoon margarine **(35)** *(f)*
- ½ cup tossed vegetable salad **(30)** *(c)* with 1 teaspoon olive oil dressing **(35)** *(f)* and lemon
- ½ cup whole milk **(75)** *(p,c,f)*

Meal 5:
- 1 peanut butter cookie **(84)** *(p,c,f)*
- 6 oz. whole milk **(112)** *(p,c,f)*

DAY 7

Meal 1:
 ½ cup cranberry-orange juice **(68)** *(c)*
 1 corn meal pancake **(68)** *(c)*
 2 teaspoons margarine **(70)** *(f)*
 1 tablespoon honey **(61)** *(c)*
 1 cup whole milk **(150)** *(p,c,f)*

Meal 2:
 1 slice whole wheat raisin bread **(60)** *(c)* covered with 1
   tablespoon peanut butter **(86)** *(p,c,f)*
 6 oz. whole milk **(112)** *(p,c,f)*
 ½ medium apple cut into wedges **(44)** *(c)*

Meal 3:
 ½ cup fish chowder **(100)** *(p,c,f)*
 ⅓ cup coleslaw **(11)** *(c)*
 ½ cup apple juice **(60)** *(c)*
 ½ oz. cheese **(55)** *(p,c,f)*
 3–4 crackers **(45)** *(c,f)*

Meal 4:
 ¼ cup fresh berries **(21)** *(c)* over ½ cup vanilla ice cream
   (145) *(p,c,f)* and topped with 2 tablespoons finely
   ground mixed nuts **(80)** *(p,f,c)*

Meal 5:
 6 oz. whole milk **(112)** *(p,c,f)*
 2 raisin cookies **(150)** *(c,f)*

DAY 8

Meal 1:

10 ripe pitted cherries (40) (c)
 1 scrambled egg (78) (p,f)
 1 slice banana bread (134) (c)
 2 teaspoons margarine (70) (f)
 ½ cup whole milk (75) (p,c,f)

Meal 2:

 1 slice whole wheat English muffin (73) (c)
 1 oz. cheese (110) (p,c,f)
 ½ cup whole milk (75) (p,c,f)

Meal 3:

CHILD'S POT ROAST:
RECIPE: Ingredients, to be placed in a pan and covered with aluminum foil then cooked in oven at 350°F for 45 minutes (or, until meat is well done), include: 1½ oz. steak (111) (p,f); ¼ sliced potato (16) (c); ¼ cup sliced carrots (11) (c). 1 tomato (22) (c)

3–4 green beans (8) (c)
 1 teaspoon margarine (35) (f)
 6 oz. whole milk (112) (p,c,f)

Meal 4:

 ½ cup cranberry juice (81) (c)
 ½ cup yogurt (75) (p,c,f) containing 1 tablespoon raisins
     (29) (c) and 2 tablespoons finely chopped almonds
     (85) (p,f,c)

Meal 5:

 1 cup whole milk (150) (p,c,f)
 1 small peach (38) (c)
 4 whole wheat crackers (64) (c,f)

DAY 9

Meal 1:

   ½ cup tomato juice **(24)** *(c)*
   ½ slice bran bread **(37)** *(c)*
   1 teaspoon margarine **(35)** *(f)*
   Poached egg **(78)** *(p,f)*

Meal 2:

   3–4 Triscuit crackers **(60)** *(c)*

   SPINACH CASSEROLE:
   RECIPE: Thaw and drain 1 10-oz. package frozen spinach. Mix
   with ½ cup canned cream of mushroom soup. Place in casserole and sprinkle with breadcrumbs. Bake 375° for 30 to 35
   minutes **(45)** *(p,f)*.
   ½ cup strawberry and melon slices **(40)** *(c)*
   1 cup whole milk **(150)** *(p,c,f)*

Meal 3:

   1½ oz. mixed seafood (flounder, striped bass, sole) **(55)** *(p)*
       cooked with ¼ cup green peppers **(8)** *(c)* and poured
       over ¼ cup rice **(41)** *(c)*
   1 teaspoon margarine **(35)** *(f)*
   ¼ cup steamed green beans **(10)** *(c)*
   ½ cup iceberg lettuce cut in shreds **(4)** *(c)*
   2 teaspoons oil **(70)** *(f)*, dash of vinegar
   1 cup whole milk **(150)** *(p,c,f)*

Meal 4:

   1 broccoli stalk **(29)** *(c)*, cooked
   2 oz. broiled ground chuck **(186)** *(p,f)*
   2 small peaches **(60)** *(c)*
   1 cup whole milk **(150)** *(p,c,f)*

Meal 5:

   ⅓ cup of pineapple and mandarin orange pieces **(40)** *(c)*,
       sprinkled with 2 tablespoons grated coconut and
       nuts **(70)** *(f)* served over ½ cup cottage cheese **(101)**
       (p,c,f)

DAY 10

Meal 1:

½ of 6-inch cantaloupe **(60)** *(c)*

FLUFFY SCRAMBLED EGG:

RECIPE: Break open an egg and separate the white and yolk. Beat white until frothy. Beat yolk until smooth. Combine white and yolk, and fry egg. **(78)** *(f,c)*

½ pumpkin muffin **(52)** *(c)*

1 teaspoon margarine **(35)** *(f)*

1 cup whole milk **(150)** *(p,c,f)*

Meal 2:

½ cup orange sections **(47)** *(c)*

CHEESE FINGERS:

RECIPE: Spread 1 teaspoon margarine **(35)** *(f)* onto one slice of oatmeal bread **(60)** *(c)*. Then place 1 oz. natural processed cheese **(107)** *(p,c,f)* onto the bread. Cut the bread into finger-width pieces and toast in oven.

1 cup whole milk **(150)** *(p,c,f)*

Meal 3:

Crunchy fruit salad: ½ cup strawberries, avocado, banana, and pineapple **(64)** *(p,c,f)*, topped with ½ cup yogurt **(75)** *(p,c,f)* and 1 teaspoon grapenuts **(12)** *(f)*

½ cup fruit juice **(64)** *(c)*

Meal 4:

½ cup vegetable soup **(58)** *(p,c)*

TOMATO VOLCANO:

RECIPE: Scoop out center of 1 tomato **(33)** *(c)* and fill with a mixture of ¼ cup salmon in oil **(91)** *(p,f)*, 2 teaspoons mayonnaise **(67)** *(f)*, and 1 teaspoon chopped celery **(6)** *(c)*.

½ cup whole milk **(75)** *(p,c,f)*

Meal 5:

1 cup whole milk **(150)** *(p,c,f)*

½ cup spinach and mushroom salad with 2 tablespoons cheese sauce **(45)** *(p,c,f)*

DAY 11

Meal 1:
> ½ cup orange slices **(47)** *(c)*
> 1 slice whole wheat raisin bread **(60)** *(c)*
> 1 cup whole milk **(150)** *(p,c,f)*

Meal 2:
> 1 hard boiled egg **(78)** *(p,f)*
> ½ slice oatmeal bread **(30)** *(c)*
> ½ cup apricot juice **(61)** *(c)*

Meal 3:
> ¼ cup fresh pineapple chunks **(17)** *(c)*
> ⅓ cup plain pudding **(110)** *(c)*
> ½ cup whole milk **(75)** *(p,c,f)*

Meal 4:
> 1½ oz. broiled steak **(111)** *(p,f)*
> ⅓ cup mashed potatoes **(60)** *(c)*
> ⅓ cup green or snow peas **(35)** *(c)*
> 1 teaspoon margarine **(35)** *(f)*
> ½ cup whole milk **(75)** *(p,c,f)*
> Fruit kabob **(40)** *(c)*: 5 small pieces of mixed fruit on a stick.

Meal 5:
> 1 cup whole milk **(150)** *(p,c,f)*
> Hand-meat pie (see page 114)

DAY 12

Meal 1:

½ banana on a stick **(42)** *(c)*
½ slice cracked wheat toast **(30)** *(c)*
1 tablespoon peanut butter **(86)** *(f)*
½ cup whole milk **(75)** *(p,c,f)*

Meal 2:

1 peanut butter cookie **(84)** *(p,c,f)*
6 oz. whole milk **(112)** *(p,c,f)*

Meal 3:

½ cup cream of chicken soup **(70)** *(c)*
1 oz. Cheddar cheese **(112)** *(p,c,f)* shredded over ½ cup
fresh fruit salad (citrus fruit and avocado) **(60)** *(p,c,f)*
½ cup grape juice **(80)** *(c)*

Meal 4:

1½ oz. roast lamb **(103)** *(p,f)*
½ cup long grain rice or barley **(79)** *(c)*
⅓ cup sweet cherries (pitted) **(40)** *(c)*
6 oz. whole milk **(112)** *(p,c,f)*

Meal 5:

1 cup whole milk **(150)** *(p,c,f)*
2 servings baked banana (African) **(200)** *(c,f)*

BAKED BANANA AFRICAN:
RECIPE: Cut 1 small, firm banana lengthwise and place in oven-proof dish. Add ½ cup water, 1 tablespoon orange juice, 1 tablespoon lemon juice, 1 teaspoon cornstarch, and 4 teaspoons margarine. Sprinkle with nutmeg. Bake at 300° for 5 to 10 minutes. Two servings, each **(100)** *(c,f)*.

DAY 13

Meal 1:
½ cup medium grapefruit sections **(30)** *(c)*
½ honey bran muffin **(58)** *(c,f)*
1 teaspoon margarine **(35)** *(f)*
1 cup whole milk **(150)** *(p,c,f)*

Meal 2:
½ cup yogurt **(75)** *(p,c,f)* mixed with 3 large strawberries
(11) *(c)* and 2 peach and pear slices **(34)** *(c)*, mashed

Meal 3:
½ slice whole wheat raisin bread **(30)** *(c)*
1 oz. natural processed cheese **(110)** *(p,c,f)*
½ cup lemonade with lime ice cubes **(51)** *(c)*

Meal 4:
1½ oz. skewered broiled ham and pineapple **(120)** *(p,f)*
¼ cup steamed rice **(41)** *(c)*
½ cup tossed green salad **(12)** *(c)*
2 tablespoons dressing **(195)** *(f)*
1 cup whole milk **(150)** *(p,c,f)*

Meal 5:
1 cup whole milk **(150)** *(p,c,f)*
2 oatmeal cookies **(160)** *(c)*
½ cup medium apple wedges **(58)** *(c)*

DAY 14

Meal 1:

½ cup orange juice **(56)** *(c)*

Cheese toast: 1 oz. natural cheese **(107)** *(p,c,f)* melted on 1 slice whole wheat bread **(56)** *(c)*

½ cup whole milk **(75)** *(p,c,f)*

Meal 2:

1 teaspoon grapenuts **(12)** *(p,c)* sprinkled over ½ cup ice cream **(139)** *(p,c,f)*

½ cup apricot juice **(61)** *(c)*

Meal 3:

¾ cup vegetable beef soup **(101)** *(c,p)*

TOMATO VOLCANO:

RECIPE: Scoop out the center of 1 tomato **(33)** *(c)* and fill with a mixture of ¼ cup tuna in oil **(96)** *(p,f)*, 3 teaspoons mayonnaise **(101)** *(f)*, and 1 teaspoon of chopped sweet pickles, celery and lettuce **(7)** *(c)*.

1 cup whole milk **(150)** *(p,c,f)*

Meal 4:

YOGURT YUM YUM:

RECIPE: ½ cup yogurt **(75)** *(p,c,f)* blended with ⅓ cup strawberries, pineapple, and banana pieces **(55)** *(c)* until stiff and again blended with 2 tablespoons finely ground nuts and coconut **(90)** *(p,c,f)*.

Meal 5:

1½ oz. meat loaf **(69)** *(p,f)*

⅓ cup steamed cabbage **(11)** *(c)*

½ small baked potato **(47)** *(c)* with 1 teaspoon margarine **(35)** *(f)*

6 oz. whole milk **(112)** *(p,f,c)*

DAY 15

Meal 1:
- ½ cup grapefruit **(30)** *(c)*
- 1 poached egg **(78)** *(p,f)*
- 1 slice whole wheat toast **(56)** *(c)*
- 1 teaspoon margarine **(35)** *(f)*
- ½ cup whole milk **(75)** *(p,c,f)*

Meal 2:
- ½ cup orange juice **(56)** *(c)*
- 2 oz. cooked beef patty, ground chuck **(186)** *(p,c,f)*
- ½ slice whole wheat bread **(28)** *(c)*
- 1 teaspoon margarine **(35)** *(f)*
- ½ cup tossed salad: tomato, lettuce, cucumber **(12)** *(c)*
- 1 teaspoon mayonnaise **(35)** *(f)*
- ½ cup spinach **(21)** *(c)*
- ½ cup whole milk **(75)** *(p,c,f)*

Meal 3:
- ¼ cup cottage cheese **(50)** *(p,c,f)*
- ½ cup fruit salad including citrus, and avocado (1 slice) **(60)** *(c,f)*
- ½ whole wheat English muffin **(73)** *(c,f)*
- 1 teaspoon margarine **(35)** *(f)*
- ½ peach **(19)** *(c)*
- ½ cup whole milk **(75)** *(p,c,f)*

Meal 4:
- 2 oz. chopped ham **(140)** *(p,c,f)*
- ½ cup steamed zucchini **(11)** *(c)*
- ½ cup steamed broccoli **(29)** *(c)*
- 2 teaspoons margarine **(70)** *(f)*
- ¼ cup crushed pineapple **(17)** *(c)*
- ½ cup whole milk **(75)** *(p,c,f)*

Meal 5:
- ½ oz. cheese **(53)** *(p,c,f)*
- ½ cup whole milk **(75)** *(p,c,f)*
- 4 wheat crackers **(64)** *(c,f)*

11

The Brain Food
Diet for Children,
Ages Four to Six

The fifteen days of menus in this chapter are
intended for children between the fourth and
sixth birthdays. As with the previous three chapters, the
foods suggested each day are balanced according to the
principles outlined in chapter seven—but here, because
of the older age of the children, approximately 1600 to
1800 calories are provided daily.

Finally, remember the abbreviations that are being
used: First, the numbers in parentheses represent the calorie values of each item. Second, the letters *p,c,f* in
parentheses indicate, respectively, whether the item is
primarily protein, carbohydrate, or fat—or a combination
of these food groups.

DAY 1

Meal 1:

    ½ cup orange sections **(47)** *(c)*

    1 bran muffin **(104)** *(c)*

    2 teaspoons margarine **(70)** *(f)*

    1 scrambled egg **(78)** *(p,f)*

    1 cup whole milk **(150)** *(p,c,f)*

Meal 2:

    1 slice raisin bread **(60)** *(c)* spread with 1½ tablespoons peanut butter **(129)** *(p,c,f)*

    ½ cup minestrone soup **(57)** *(c)*

    ½ cup whole milk **(75)** *(p,c,f)*

Meal 3:

    1 oz. ham **(70)** *(p,f)* and 1 oz. brie cheese **(94)** *(p,f)* in ½ piece Syrian pocket bread **(68)** *(c)*

    3 slices of tomato **(10)** *(c)* and ⅓ cup flower pieces of raw cauliflower **(10)** *(c)*

    6 oz. whole milk **(112)** *(p,c,f)*

Meal 4:

    ½ cup whole milk **(75)** *(p,c,f)*

    ⅓ cup mashed potatoes **(60)** *(c)*

    2 oz. roast chicken **(70)** *(p)*

    ½ cup green peas **(55)** *(c)*

    2 teaspoons margarine **(70)** *(f)*

    ½ cup frozen fruit juice on a stick **(64)** *(c)*

Meal 5:

    1 cup whole milk **(150)** *(p,c,f)*

    1 peanut butter cookie **(84)** *(p,c,f)*

DAY 2

Meal 1:

    ½ cup cantaloupe and watermelon pieces **(26)** *(c)*
    1 soya muffin **(119)** *(c)*
    2 teaspoons margarine **(70)** *(f)*
    1 cup whole milk **(150)** *(p,c,f)*

Meal 2:

    ROAST BEEF SANDWICH:
RECIPE: 1 thin slice roast beef **(93)** *(p,f)* on 1 slice whole wheat bread **(56)** *(c)*, spread with 1 tablespoon mayonnaise **(101)** *(f)* and topped by 1 lettuce leaf and 1 slice tomato **(10)** *(c)*

    1 carrot stick **(20)** *(c)*
    ½ cup split-pea soup **(104)** *(p,c)*
    1 cup whole milk **(150)** *(p,c,f)*

Meal 3:

    ½ cup whole milk **(75)** *(p,c,f)*
    1 slice raisin bread **(60)** *(c)*
    1½ tablespoons peanut butter **(128)** *(p,c,f)*

Meal 4:

    ½ cup macaroni and cheese **(205)** *(p,f)*
    2 tomato slices **(10)** *(c)*
    1 raw apple **(87)** *(c)*
    6 oz. whole milk **(112)** *(p,c,f)*

Meal 5:

    1 oz. natural cheese **(107)** *(p,c,f)*
    4 whole wheat crackers **(64)** *(c)*
    1 cup fruit juice **(129)** *(c)*

DAY 3

Meal 1:

2 small apricots **(40)** *(c)*

CHINESE OMELET:
RECIPE: Separate egg white from yolk. Beat white until it stands in peaks. Beat egg yolk until thick. Stir in a pinch of salt and 1 tablespoon of finely chopped cooked snow peas and broccoli. Fold mixture into egg whites. Use 2 teaspoons margarine to cook in hot skillet; turn only once. **(150)** *(p,c,f)*

1 slice rye bread **(56)** *(c)*
2 teaspoons margarine **(70)** *(f)*
1 cup whole milk **(150)** *(p,c,f)*

Meal 2:

PEANUT BUTTER/CHEESE SANDWICH:
RECIPE: 1 slice raisin bread **(60)** *(c)* spread with 1 tablespoon peanut butter **(86)** *(p,f)*, topped with 1 oz. natural cheese **(107)** *(p,c,f)* and toasted.

10 large strawberries **(37)** *(c)*
½ cup whole milk **(75)** *(p,c,f)*

Meal 3:

½ cup cottage cheese **(101)** *(p,c,f)*, covered with ½ cup raw cauliflower, broccoli, green pepper, celery, and carrots **(20)** *(c)* finely cut
½ cup pineapple juice **(50)** *(c)*

Meal 4:

1 serving salmon loaf **(119)** *(p,c,f)*
2 teaspoons margarine **(70)** *(f)*
½ cup steamed cabbage with lemon **(16)** *(c)*
1 cup tossed salad leaves **(20)** *(c)*
1 tablespoon Italian dressing **(77)** *(f)*
½ cup melon **(26)** *(c)*
½ cup whole milk **(75)** *(p,c,f)*

Meal 5:

1 cup whole milk **(150)** *(p,c,f)*
3 Graham crackers **(81)** *(c)*

DAY 4

Meal 1:

- ½ cup grapefruit (41) (c)
- ½ cup hot oatmeal (74) (c), topped with 2 teaspoons margarine (70) (f)
- 1 cup whole milk (150) (p,c,f)

Meal 2:

- ½ cup applesauce (41) (c)
- 3 whole wheat crackers (48) (c)
- 1 tablespoon peanut butter (86) (p,f,c)
- ½ cup whole milk (75) (p,c,f)

Meal 3:

CRAB CASSEROLE:
RECIPE: Mix 1 cup crabmeat (drained and with cartilage removed), 4 mushrooms (finely chopped), 1 gherkin (finely diced), ½ teaspoon pimiento (finely chopped), 1 teaspoon chopped parsley, and 1 teaspoon chopped onion. Melt 2 table-spoons margarine, and add 3 tablespoons all-purpose flour. Boil 1 cup milk and stir into margarine/flour mixture with a whisk. Add ⅛ teaspoon salt. Mix crabmeat mixture with sauce and pour into greased casserole. Sprinkle with breadcrumbs and bake at 350° for 30 minutes. Garnish with 1 or 2 pimiento-stuffed olives (optional). Serve ⅓ cup. (100) (p,c,f)

- ¾ cup raisin-carrot salad: ½ cup grated carrots (22) (c), 2 tablespoons raisins (58) (c), and 1 tablespoon mayonnaise (101) (f)
- 1 small plum (22) (c)
- 1 cup whole milk (150) (p,c,f)

Meal 4:

- ¾ cup chili (180) (p,c,f)
- 1 small slice corn bread (105) (c)
- 1 teaspoon margarine (35) (f)
- 6 oz. whole milk (112) (p,c,f)
  Fruit kabob (40) (c): 5 small pieces of mixed fruit on a stick

Meal 5:

- ¾ cup fruit salad: strawberry, avocado, and pineapple (63) (p,c,f)
- 2 oatmeal cookies (160) (c)
- ½ cup fruit juice (64) (c)

DAY 5

Meal 1:

>½ cup orange juice (**56**) *(c)*
>Chicken-liver omelet: 1 tablespoon chicken-liver
>   shavings mixed with 1 egg (**140**) *(p,c,f)*
>1 corn muffin (**130**) *(c)*
>2 teaspoons margarine (**70**) *(f)*
>1 cup whole milk (**150**) *(p,c,f)*

Meal 2:

>½ cup vegetable (bean) soup (**55**) *(p,c)*
>3 whole wheat crackers (**48**) *(c)*
>1 small apple (**40**) *(c)*
>6 oz. whole milk (**112**) *(p,f,c)*

Meal 3:

>½ cup apple juice (**60**) *(c)*

TUNA SALAD PLATE:
RECIPE: 1 tomato (**22**) *(c)*, cut into small pieces, and mixed with
¼ cup tuna fish in oil (**96**) *(p,f)* and 1 tablespoon mayonnaise
(**101**) *(f)*, 1 teaspoon green pepper, and onion and celery finely
diced (**8**) *(c)*

>½ cup ice cream (**139**) *(p,c,f)*

Meal 4:

>2 oz. broiled veal (**132**) *(p)*
>½ cup carrot and pineapple salad (**60**) *(c)*
>6 oz. whole milk (**112**) *(p,c,f)*

Meal 5:

>1 bran muffin (**104**) *(c)*
>1 tablespoon peanut butter (**86**) *(p,c,f)*
>½ cup whole milk (**75**) *(p,c,f)*

DAY 6

Meal 1:

½ cup apricot juice (**61**) (c)
1 slice peanut butter raisin bread (**75**) (c)
1 teaspoon margarine (**35**) (f)
1 cup whole milk (**150**) (p,c,f)

Meal 2:

¾ cup fish chowder (**150**) (p,c,f)
5–6 whole wheat crackers (**88**) (c)
½ cup coleslaw (with mayonnaise, lemon, and vinegar)
(**86**) (c,f)
1 small apple cut in wedges (**40**) (c)
1 cup whole milk (**150**) (p,c,f)

Meal 3:

Pocket sandwich: 2 oz. ground beef (**186**) (p,f) in ½ medium
size Syrian pocket bread (**68**) (c)
⅓ cup celery and carrot sticks (**10**) (c)
½ cup frozen fruit juice on a stick (**64**) (c)
6 oz. whole milk (**112**) (p,c,f)

Meal 4:

¼ cup beef ravioli (**150**) (p,c,f)
½ cup stewed tomatoes (**26**) (c)
½ cup mixed salad leaves (**15**) (c)
2 teaspoons oil (**70**) (f)
½ cup peach/pear/apricot juice (**62**) (c)

Meal 5:

¾ cup yogurt (**112**) (p,f,c), mixed with 1 tablespoon
almond slivers and coconut flakes (**48**) (p,c,f), and 1
teaspoon raisins (**13**) (c)

DAY 7

Meal 1:

    1 hard boiled egg **(78)** *(p,f)*
    ½ corn muffin **(65)** *(c)*
    1 teaspoon margarine **(35)** *(f)*
    ½ cup whole milk **(75)** *(p,c,f)*

Meal 2:

    ½ cup lentil soup **(130)** *(p,c)*
    ½ slice raisin bread **(30)** *(c)*
    1 tablespoon peanut butter **(86)** *(p,c,f)*
    ½ cup apple juice **(60)** *(c)*

Meal 3:

    1 oz. natural cheese **(107)** *(p,f)*, shredded over 1 cup fresh
        fruit salad: citrus fruits and avocado **(145)** *(c,f)*
    ½ whole wheat muffin **(50)** *(c)*, spread with 2 teaspoons
        margarine **(70)** *(f)*
    1 wedge of tomato **(10)** *(c)* and ½ cucumber, sliced **(10)**
        (c), both garnished with 2 teaspoons oil, **(70)** *(f)* and
        sprig of mint and dash of vinegar
    6 oz. of whole milk **(112)** *(p,c,f)*

Meal 4:

    STEAK ITALIAN:
RECIPE: Broil 1½ oz. steak **(111)** *(p,f)* with ½ tomato **(20)** *(c)* and
½ cup mushroom slices **(10)** *(c)* and pour over ¼ cup spaghetti
(45) *(c)*. Top with 4 teaspoons grated cheese **(110)** *(p,c,f)*.
    ½ cup chopped uncooked spinach **(14)** *(c)* mixed with 1
        tablespoon Italian dressing **(77)** *(f)*
    ½ cup orange juice **(56)** *(c)*

Meal 5:

    6 oz. whole milk **(112)** *(p,c,f)*
    10 seedless grapes **(25)** *(c)*

DAY 8

Meal 1:
- ½ cup blueberries **(43)** *(c)*
- 1 oatmeal muffin **(104)** *(c)*
- 2 teaspoons margarine **(70)** *(f)*
- 1 scrambled egg **(78)** *(p,f)*
- 1 cup whole milk **(150)** *(p,c,f)*

Meal 2:
- ½ cup whole milk **(75)** *(p,c,f)*
- ⅓ cup mashed potatoes **(60)** *(c)*
- 1½ oz. roast pork **(139)** *(p,f)*
- ½ cup green peas **(53)** *(c)*
- 2½ teaspoons margarine **(88)** *(f)*
- 1 pineapple slice and teaspoon of juice **(50)** *(c)* sprinkled with 1 tablespoon raisins **(29)** *(c)*

Meal 3:
- 3–4 Triscuit crackers **(73)** *(c)*
- 1½ tablespoons peanut butter **(129)** *(p,c)*
- ½ cup minestrone soup **(57)** *(c)*
- ½ cup whole milk **(75)** *(p,c,f)*

Meal 4:

CORN AND TONGUE CASSEROLE:
RECIPE: Blend 2¼ cups of whole kernel corn with ¾ cup whole milk, ¾ cup dried bread crumbs, 1 teaspoon chopped onion, and 1 teaspoon chopped green pepper. Add corn mixture and ½ cup thinly sliced tongue in alternate layers into greased casserole. Sprinkle 2 tablespoons dried bread crumbs and 1 teaspoon finely chopped parsley over the top; then dot with 3 teaspoons margarine. Cook in oven at 350 for 30-45 minutes. **(273)** *(p,c,f)*
- ⅓ cup carrots **(15)** *(c)*
- 1 cup zucchini and yellow squash, raw and slivered with grater or food processor **(20)** *(c)*
- 1 tablespoon Italian dressing **(77)** *(f)*
- ½ cup whole milk **(75)** *(p,c,f)*

Meal 5:
- 1 cup whole milk **(150)** *(p,c,f)*
- 1 peanut butter cookie **(84)** *(p,c,f)*

DAY 9

Meal 1:

   1½ tangerines in pieces **(60)** *(c)*
   1 deviled egg **(145)** *(p,f)*
   1 cup whole milk **(150)** *(p,c,f)*
   3 rye crackers **(72)** *(c,f)*

Meal 2:

   ½ cup orange-pineapple juice **(60)** *(c)*

   TUNA SANDWICH:
   RECIPE: 1 slice whole wheat bread **(56)** *(c)*, spread with ½ cup tuna in oil **(192)** *(p,f)*, mixed with 3 teaspoons mayonnaise **(101)** *(f)* and dash of lemon juice, 1 thinly sliced pickle, and 1 lettuce leaf **(8)** *(c)*.

Meal 3:

   2 oz. broiled chicken **(70)** *(p,f)*, cooked with 2 teaspoons
      margarine **(70)** *(f)*
   1 cup fresh green beans **(40)** *(c)*
   1 cup salad: cucumber, tomato, lettuce, avocado **(140)**
      (p,c,f) with 2 teaspoons oil **(70)** *(f)* and dash of
      vinegar
   1 cup whole milk **(150)** *(p,c,f)*

Meal 4:

   ½ cup baked lima beans **(40)** *(p,f)*, covered with 2
      tablespoons bread-crumbs **(25)** *(c)*
   ½ cup strawberries and banana slices **(45)** *(c)*
   ½ cup whole milk **(75)** *(p,c,f)*

Meal 5:

   ½ cup of ice cream **(139)** *(p,c,f)*, topped with 2
      tablespoons dates, prunes, figs (dried) **(40)** *(c)*
   ½ cup cranberry juice **(81)** *(c)*

DAY 10

Meal 1:

½ cup fresh grapefruit sections (**30**) *(c)*

½ cup hot oatmeal (**74**) *(c)*, cooked with 2 teaspoons
margarine (**70**) *(f)*

1 cup whole milk (**150**) *(p,c,f)*

Meal 2:

Fruit salad: ½ tangerine, 5 grapes (seedless), 1 apple wedge
(**60**) *(c)*

3 whole wheat crackers (**48**) *(c)*

1 tablespoon peanut butter (**86**) *(p,c,f)*

½ cup whole milk (**75**) *(p,c,f)*

Meal 3:

YOK YOUNG STIR-FRIED MEAL:

RECIPE: Use 3 teaspoons oil (**105**) *(f)* in a wok or deep frying
pan to stir and fry ¾ cup mixed vegetables, including snow
peas, onions, mushrooms, carrots, chopped broccoli, bamboo
shoots, celery, and water chestnuts (**81**) *(c)*. To this mixture add
2 oz. cooked chopped (chuck) beef (**186**) *(p,f)* and 1 teaspoon
powered almonds (**45**) *(p,c,f)*. Serve over ½ cup brown rice (**89**)
(c) and season with 2 teaspoons soy sauce.

½ cup orange juice (**56**) *(c)*

Meal 4:

2 oz. corned beef (**186**) *(p,f)*

½ cup steamed cabbage (**16**) *(c)*

1 slice Irish soda bread (**70**) *(c)*

2 teaspoons margarine (**70**) *(f)*

6 oz. whole milk (**112**) *(p,c,f)*

Meal 5:

¾ cup fruit: strawberry, avocado, pineapple (**95**) *(p,c,f)*

2 tablespoons plain yogurt (**19**) *(p,c,f)*

½ cup whole milk (**75**) *(p,c,f)*

DAY 11

Meal 1:

1 raisin bun (**62**) *(c,f)*
2 teaspoons margarine (**70**) *(f)*
½ cup berries (**43**) *(c)*
1 cup whole milk (**150**) *(p,c,f)*

Meal 2:

½ cup whole milk (**75**) *(p,c,f)*
1 slice corn bread (**105**) *(c)*
1½ tablespoons peanut butter (**129**) *(p,c,f)*

Meal 3:

1½ oz. chicken liver (**90**) *(p,f)*, sautéed in 2 teaspoons
    margarine (**70**) *(f)*
1 ear corn (**100**) *(c)*
½ cup tossed vegetable salad: lettuce and spinach (**10**) *(c)*
    Dressing: 2 teaspoons sweet oil (**70**) *(f)* and dash of
    vinegar
½ cup whole milk (**75**) *(p,c,f)*

Meal 4:

½ cup tangerine juice (**54**) *(c)*

TURKEY SANDWICH:
RECIPE: 1 slice cracked wheat bread (**60**) *(c)*, 1 oz. thinly sliced
turkey (**54**) *(p)*, 1 tablespoon mayonnaise (**101**) *(f)*, 1 lettuce leaf
and 1 slice tomato (**10**) *(c)*
1 carrot stick (**20**) *(c)*
¼ cup bean salad: green, wax, kidney (**15**) *(p,c)*
    Dressing: 1 teaspoon oil (**35**) *(f)* with dash of vinegar
1 cup whole milk (**150**) *(p,c,f)*

Meal 5:

½ cup whole milk (**75**) *(p,c,f)*
½ avocado (**127**) *(f,c)* mashed and mixed with 1 teaspoon
    Italian dressing (**26**) *(f)*, on 1–2 whole wheat crackers
    (**24**) *(c)*

DAY 12

Meal 1:

    ½ cup melon **(26)** *(c)*
    1 egg **(78)** *(p,f)* fried in 2 teaspoons margarine **(70)** *(f)*
    1 slice oatmeal bread **(60)** *(c)*
    ½ cup whole milk **(75)** *(p,c,f)*

Meal 2:

    BUNK HOUSE FARE:

RECIPE: 1½ oz. broiled steak pieces **(111)** *(p,f)* cooked with ¼ cup mushrooms and tomato **(100)** *(p,f)*, served on ¼ cup cartwheel or wagonwheel pasta **(45)** *(c)*

    ½ cup spinach salad **(15)** *(c)*, with 1 tablespoon Italian
        dressing **(77)** *(f)*
    1 fresh nectarine **(32)** *(c)*
    6 oz. whole milk **(112)** *(p,c,f)*

Meal 3:

    ¾ cup lentil soup **(195)** *(p,c)*
    ½ cup fresh fruit salad (include avocado and citrus fruit)
        (60) *(c,f)*
    ½ whole wheat muffin **(50)** *(c)*
    1 teaspoon margarine **(35)** *(f)*
    1 tomato wedge **(10)** *(c)*
    Sliced cucumber **(10)** *(c)*, with 2 teaspoons oil and dash
        of vinegar **(70)** *(f)*
    1 cup whole milk **(150)** *(p,c,f)*

Meal 4:

    ½ cup ice cream **(139)** *(p,c,f)*
    1 tablespoon granola **(10)** *(c)*, with 1 tablespoon raisins
        (20) *(c)*

Meal 5:

    1 cup whole milk **(150)** *(p,c,f)*
    ½ banana on a stick **(42)** *(c)*

DAY 13

Meal 1:

> ½ cup orange juice (**56**) *(c)*
> 1 slice French toast (**119**) *(p,c,f)*
> 2 teaspoons margarine (**70**) *(f)*
> 6 oz. milk (**112**) *(p,c,f)*

Meal 2:

> ½ cup yogurt (**75**) *(p,c,f)*, with ⅓ cup avocado (**40**) *(c,f)*
>   blended in
> ½ cup apricot juice (**61**) *(c)*

Meal 3:

> 2 oz. deviled beef (**138**) *(p,f)*
> ¼ cup seasoned green peas (**27**) *(c)*
> 1 cup tossed green salad (**24**) *(c)*
> 1 tablespoon Italian dressing (**77**) *(f)*
> ½ cup watermelon (**26**) *(c)*
> ½ cup whole milk (**75**) *(p,c,f)*

Meal 4:

Peanut butter/cheese sandwich: 1 slice raisin bread (**60**) *(c)*,
spread with 1 tablespoon peanut butter (**86**) *(p,f)* and 1 oz.
natural cheese (**107**) *(p,c,f)*
> 10 large strawberries (**37**) *(c)*
> 6 oz. whole milk (**112**) *(p,c,f)*

Meal 5:

> 6 oz. whole milk (**112**) *(p,c,f)*
> 2 oatmeal raisin cookies (**126**) *(c,f)*

DAY 14

Meal 1:

    3 orange wedges (**23**) *(c)*
    2 Creole *bagnets* (French fruit fritters) (**95**) *(c,f)*
    1 cup whole milk (**150**) *(p,c,f)*

Meal 2:

    TOMATO VOLCANO:

RECIPE: Scoop out pulp of 1 tomato (**20**) *(c)*, mix with ¼ cup tuna fish in oil (**96**) *(p,f)* and 1 tablespoon mayonnaise (**101**) *(f)*; add 1 teaspoon chopped sweet pickle and celery (**8**) *(c)* and return mixture to tomato shell.

    1 pear in slices (**100**) *(c)*
    1 cup whole milk (**150**) *(p,c,f)*

Meal 3:

    ½ cup vegetable (bean) soup (**55**) *(p,c)*
    3 whole wheat crackers (**48**) *(c)*
    2 teaspoons margarine (**70**) *(f)*
    ½ cup whole milk (**75**) *(p,c,f)*

Meal 4:

    2 oz. boiled chicken (**70**) *(p)*
    Cooked broccoli spear (**29**) *(c)*, with 1 teaspoon
        margarine (**35**) *(f)*
    ½ cup brown rice (**89**) *(c)*
    1 cup whole milk (**150**) *(p,c,f)*

Meal 5:

    YOGURT YUM-YUM:

RECIPE: 1 cup yogurt (**150**) *(p,c,f)*, mixed in blender with ½ cup strawberry, pear, and banana pieces (**81**) *(c)*. Add 3 tablespoons finely ground mixed nuts and coconut (**135**) *(p,c,f)*.

DAY 15

Meal 1:
>½ cup orange juice **(56)** *(c)*
>½ cup oats and wheat **(80)** *(p,c,f)*
>1 whole wheat toast slice **(56)** *(c)*
>1 cup whole milk **(150)** *(p,c,f)*

Meal 2:
>½ cup fruit salad **(43)** *(c,f)*, including ½ slice avocado
>1 biscuit **(130)** *(c,f)*
>½ cup whole milk **(75)** *(p,c,f)*

Meal 3:
>2 oz. slice turkey **(108)** *(p)*
>1 slice whole wheat bread **(56)** *(c)*
>2 teaspoons margarine **(70)** *(f)*
>½ cup cooked broccoli **(29)** *(c)*
>½ cup cooked cauliflower **(12)** *(c)*
>½ cup whole milk **(75)** *(p,c,f)*
>1 medium pear **(100)** *(c)*, topped with ¼ cup cottage
>   cheese **(50)** *(c,p,f)*

Meal 4:
>2 oz. round steak **(148)** *(p,c,f)*
>2 teaspoons margarine **(70)** *(f)*
>½ cup lettuce, cucumber and tomato **(20)** *(c)*
>½ cup Sight Savers Salad **(30)** *(c)* (see page 114)
>1 small apple **(50)** *(c)*
>1 small boiled ear of corn **(100)** *(c)*
>1 teaspoon margarine **(35)** *(f)*
>½ cup whole milk **(75)** *(p,c,f)*
>½ cup watermelon **(26)** *(c)*

Meal 5:
>½ cup fresh strawberries **(28)** *(c)*
>1 oz. cheese **(107)** *(p,f)*
>1 whole wheat cracker **(16)** *(c)*
>1 cup whole milk **(150)** *(p,c,f)*

12

Food Strategies
for Finicky
Preschoolers

Now that you know which foods will promote healthy brain development—and you have menus laid out for you—you might think the rest would be easy. But as the parent of a young child, you're well aware that the fight has only begun. Knowing what foods your youngster should eat is relatively easy compared to the problem of getting that brain food into the mouth and down into the stomach.

Preschoolers are notorious for being finicky eaters. There are a number of good reasons for this trait. First of all, their growth rate is slower than it was in infancy, and so they don't require as much food as they did earlier in life. Also, they're just "trying out their wings"—walking, talking, and testing the limits their parents have placed on them. The war of the wills has begun, and the meal table is often the primary battleground.

Despite the variety of good reasons for the child's resistance to eating on command, this period of life is critical for brain development. That is why I'm including the following feeding strategies to help you in your ongoing effort to get that preschooler to finish his meals.

Strategy Number One:
Analyze Your Child's Eating Cycle

If you're nervous or uneasy about what your child is eating, he'll pick up on your anxiety and will probably respond in the opposite way to what you want. Remember: Your child won't be as hungry in the later preschool years as he was during the first eighteen months. Also, because the child is becoming more independent between age two and five, he is likely to rebel if you continually push food at him.

So don't set yourself up for a conflict. All appetites are variable, and sometimes a child just doesn't feel like eating the food set before him. Instead, do what you can do about getting your child to eat, and be as creative as you possibly can. You may change the place of eating from the kitchen to the dining room; or you may have a picnic on a blanket indoors. You can even take a lunch to the playground, to the zoo, or on other outings. If nothing seems to work, see your pediatrician for specific counseling about your child's problem.

Strategy Number Two:
Avoid the Three-Meals-a-Day Trap

This strategy reflects my belief in the need for about five meals a day for infants, toddlers, and preschoolers.

Obviously, you can't always be prepared for a child's moment of hunger. But if you're out on a trip, you might pack a nutritious lunch or snack—one of your "five meals"—so that you won't have to go to the nearest junk food outlet to satisfy his demands.

Strategy Number Three:
Let Your Child Be the Chef

I'm not talking about putting the youngster next to the stove, of course. But let him help you make sandwiches, salads, or anything else that's simple and safe. Also, the child may enjoy setting the table, selecting where family members will sit, clearing the dishes off after the meal, or otherwise participating in the preparation and clean-up.

For some reason—perhaps because of the increasing need for some control over their environment—children are more likely to eat their food if they helped prepare it. Preschool programs for children often rely heavily on this principle.

Strategy Number Four:
There's No Such Thing as a
"Yukky" Food

Mealtime should be a marvelous social experience. The child can see how the mother, the father, and the rest of the family interact: he can see how they eat, and observe their relationship to food and to each other. So it's important to provide your preschooler with this valuable aspect of socialization.

One word of caution, however: Keep in mind that the youngster will imitate older members of the family. If someone says "yuk" to a certain food, don't expect the preschooler observing this reaction to be enthusiastic about the dish either. This becomes all the more of a problem if the negative response has been directed toward one of the child's brain foods.

So be a good model, and encourage others in the family to behave likewise. Try to direct conversations away from negative comments about the kind of food on the table or the style of the preschooler's eating habits because either may dampen the youngster's appetite.

Strategy Number Five:
Honor the "Grown-Up" Instinct

Between six months and five years of age, the child moves from a dependent position to an independent one. He gradually starts wanting to do many things for himself, including feeding himself.

It's important to let this development take place naturally. You may find, for example, at times when your child wants to feed himself and you try to do it for him because you're more efficient, he'll refuse the food altogether. So, don't take away his motivation and emerging independence, thus setting the stage for conflict at the dinner table. Rather, if he wants to feed himself, let him—even if he prefers to use his fingers or occasionally spills food on the table or the floor.

Realize at the start of this process that it's going to be messy, and prepare. An oil cloth on the floor under the child's chair can take much of the parental anxiety out of impending messiness. If you don't allow your child to feed himself when he's ready, you'll be thwarting his desire to be independent, and he may end up rejecting his food completely.

In this messy stage, by the way, it's helpful to focus on foods he can pick up with his fingers, such as cheese, soft breads, lightly cooked carrots, tender chicken, and chunks of tuna.

Finally, remember the other side of the coin during this stage of emerging independence: Your youngster may want to be independent at mealtimes, but he may then become distracted and lose interest. It's important for you to step in and continue the feeding in such cases—even at what you may consider to be a relatively advanced age. For example, if your two-and-a-half or three year old refuses to feed himself through most meals and you see other children of a similar age wielding forks and spoons with great aplomb, don't worry! Remember: The key thing is to get that brain food down into his stomach! He can learn the fine art of feeding himself after his brain is fully formed.

Strategy Number Six:
Don't Be Afraid to Try the "Toy Trick"

The personal maturity that is necessary for perfect table manners may not develop completely in most children until about age five. As a result, no matter how hard you try to teach dining skills, you may very well fail until the child has gotten a little older.

For example, children may want to "feed" their toy animals or dolls as they eat, and my feeling is that this is a perfectly acceptable practice. I know one family that has discovered their three-year-old eats just fine as long as he has a couple of his toys on the table and his mother or father is feeding him half the time as he plays with them.

Some parents might feel that such practices promote bad habits. I've seen too many children, however, who don't eat properly because they have resisted their parents' ideas about the right thing to do at the table. When a child is frustrated, there's less chance that he's going to eat enough of the foods that will help his brain to develop properly.

Strategy Number Seven:
Let Your Child Play "Eating"

One of the things that may prevent your child from eating his brain food—especially in the first two years of life—is the fact that he will probably enjoy playing with it with his fingers more than putting it into his mouth. And why shouldn't he? Putting things in a cup, pouring them out, watching juice run all over the place—these are rather exciting and intriguing pastimes to a youngster. Chances are, mealtime is the only time he gets to see and play with such interesting toys.

For this reason, I recommend that you provide your child with cups and liquids at playtime, as well as at mealtime. This way, when you sit your child down to eat, playing with the food will be less of a novelty and he'll be more likely to concentrate on eating.

Strategy Number Eight:
Bribes Don't Go Well with Brain Food

Almost every parent uses bribes or the threat of punishment to a certain extent to get their children to eat.

Often, we aren't even aware of what we're doing! For example, have you ever caught yourself saying, "No cake until you finish your vegetables"? Or how many times have you said, 'Don't be a bad boy! Sit there until you finish your milk!" There's also the familiar guilt ploy, "Now, think of all the starving children in the world!" Or, perhaps worst of all, "If you don't behave, you'll have to go to bed without your dinner!"

Finally, how many times have you gone to a doctor's—or even a dentist's—office, and witnessed your child receive a lollipop as a reward?

While tactics like these may work in terms of persuading a child to calm down or behave better, they establish poor eating habits and may cause him to miss out on important nutrients for his brain development. A junk-food bribe almost always becomes a substitute for one or more of the five meals a day your child should be eating. If you want to reward or punish your child, use other methods—but not food!

Strategy Number Nine:
A Child Shouldn't Starve for
Lack of Table Skills

Sometimes a youngster may balk at eating, not because of the food that's available, but because of the technique or skill that his parents require of him. For example, if you put your child's milk into a large glass, it may be that he can't comfortably hold the container. Changing to a small cup with two handles might make all the difference in the world. Remember: The myelination or sheathing of brain cells that probably controls coordination is still taking place up to about age five.

Similarly, don't fill the cup with more than the child

can safely manage. A full cup may look overwhelming to a two year old, while a half-filled container that contains a couple of swallows may seem just right.

One important point here is that you should become keenly aware of your child's motor skills—of what he or she can and cannot accomplish physically. Above all, don't use mealtimes as a training ground for fine motor skills at the expense of too little food!

Finally, your child should be comfortable and safe at the table. Choose a high chair, booster seat, or some other seating arrangement with this principle in mind.

Strategy Number Ten:
Always Announce Mealtimes in Advance

Interrupting your child's favorite activity to eat, without prior notice, is asking for trouble. Like you, your child will tend to get quite involved in his "work" and play. If you snatch him up to eat right in the middle of a fascinating game with his trucks or blocks, you're asking for conflict. The youngster will resent the intrusion and probably blame you, and the food as well, for spoiling his fun.

So give your youngster some advance warning. You'd be surprised at how well even very young children two years old or even younger, respond to and understand an explanation of what's coming up and what's expected of them. I would suggest that you let your children know at least ten minutes in advance that lunch is almost ready so they can begin to wind up their activities. Then, remind them again with five minutes to go and do so again one minute before it's time to sit down at the table.

Strategy Number Eleven:
Set Time Limits

If your child tends to be a lollygagger, taking forty-five minutes or more to eat, here's what you can do. Reduce the amount of time devoted to eating each day, a small increment at a time, until you reach the ideal time period. Give him periodic notice that it's important to finish up because he has other fun things waiting for him to do.

But under no circumstances should you deliver a fiat such as "Mealtime will last thirty minutes, and that's it!" Remember: Your child wants some independence, and such an effort to control him completely at mealtimes will make him less inclined to eat properly.

Strategy Number Twelve:
Select Preschool Table Settings

At a very young age, adult forks and spoons just don't work properly in little hands. There are many utensils on the market today which are perfect for your child's fingers. You might shop around and find the combination that seems to work best at a given age.

One thing I particularly recommend you *not* use, at least for children under three, is the adult fork. Seeing a child wave a fork in the air can create a great deal of tension in a parent. Any time this happens, the youngster will be less likely to eat well.

So, use a spoon or a small, dull child's fork. A spoon works just as well for a child as a fork, if not better. It's certainly safer, is likely to cause less anxiety, and is therefore conducive to a more pleasurable eating environment.

Strategy Number Thirteen:
Don't Strike Out When You Eat Out

It's fine to take your two year old out for dinner. But make sure the restaurant has his brain foods on the menu, as well as the proper environment to entice him to eat properly.

For example, be sure you can get to the restaurant before it gets too near to his bedtime or past his usual mealtime, and he becomes cranky or sleepy. Check how long the wait for a table will be, too. Even the best-trained five year old may be unable to stand in a line for very long without misbehaving.

Also, you should see how close the tables are to one another. If they're within reaching distance, your youngster may be tempted to play with the clothing or other accoutrements of those at neighboring tables.

Finally, check to see how long it takes the restaurant to serve meals. A long, leisurely meal may be great for the romantic adult but decidedly the opposite for a hungry, impatient child.

Strategy Number Fourteen:
Establish Your Authority

This certainly doesn't mean you should be a drill sergeant or interfere unnecessarily with your child's need for independence. But is does mean that you should set certain limits, and decide what's going to happen if the boy or girl exceeds those limits.

For example, it's obviously unacceptable to throw food around; to hit other family members with eating utensils; or to refuse to come to the table unless the entire table is covered with toys. Establish your eating policies and priorities in advance, inform the child of your intentions, and build a certain amount of flexibility into your plan. But do be ready to crack down with a stern word or non-food-related punishment if your child pushes you too far. One important principle to keep in mind is that the parents should present a united front. If one says, "Stop that," and the other says, "Oh, it's all right," the child will get mixed signals and is likely to obey neither.

Finally, keep your top priority in mind: The key consideration over the long haul is getting those brain foods into your child's stomach. Discipline is essential to a child's social development, but try as hard as you can to keep your mealtimes relaxed and punishment-free.

Strategy Number Fifteen:
A Child Is Never Too Young for
a Course in Good Nutrition

Tell your child why he should eat certain foods, even if he seems uninterested in your explanations. A lot more than we sometimes realize sinks into those developing young minds. To encourage the learning process, it's helpful to use props and draw graphic word pictures as you try to get your points across.

For example, as you do your calisthenics in the morning, you might discuss how strong muscles are formed by exercise *and* nutrition. Also, talk about what different kinds of food can do for different functions of the body. Fruit and vegetables, you might say, are "super-foods" (you might even say they're "complex carbohydrates" and have him repeat the words), which provide quick energy and help him run faster and longer distances.

Strategy Number Sixteen:
Make Eating an Adventure

Children, like adults, will begin to center on their favorite foods and ask for them frequently. This kind of natural selection process is fine, especially if the foods the child likes are brain foods. But it's also important to get the child introduced at an early age to new dishes so that he'll have a wide variety of brain foods to choose from in case one of his favorites is unavailable.

One way to do this is to put the new food into something the child already likes. For example, my own son's favorite food for a time was squash. To get him used to eating unfamiliar items, we introduced a complete array of foods into his squash—such as veal and peas. This way, he learned to enjoy the new flavors in combination with a proven "winner."

Strategy Number Seventeen:
Variety Is the Spice of Life for a Successful Brain Food Diet

Just because your child doesn't like a fried egg, that doesn't mean he won't like it scrambled, hard-boiled, or deviled. The problem may be the appearance or consistency of the food; his resistance may have nothing to do with the taste. So, if he won't eat a certain food one way, try fixing it another and another until you find exactly the right formula.

Also, always try to make the food look attractive and feel interesting. Children are very sensitive to food textures. In the second year, as more teeth appear, your child will welcome more chewable food. So, instead of

trying to feed him something like applesauce, which he
may have liked a year earlier, try shredding an apple or
baking it to give it a different, more chewable texture.

Simple, colorful foods—those, for instance, that are
red, green, or white—are attractive to children. Mushy,
unidentifiable food tends to be unappetizing. Extremely
hot or cold foods can be frightening or dangerous. Adult
amounts of food may seem overwhelming to a child, so
you might experiment with varying portions until you
find the right size serving.

Now you should have all of the brain food "ammuni-
tion" you need to get your child off on the right track.
You know the proper foods, and you know how to serve
them; in addition, you have a complete set of sample
menus. The time has finally come to launch your own
Brain Food Diet for your child.

But before you begin—and before I end this book—I
want to leave one final thought with you: Above all, after
you've settled on an intelligent brain food program,
relax! An anxiety-ridden parent often creates many more
problems than are generated by a few mistakes in a basi-
cally well-designed dietary program. So do your best;
love your child; and *enjoy* the experience as you watch
the marvelous potential of a young mind unfold before
your eyes.

Bibliography

American Academy of Pediatrics, Committee on Nutrition. "Vitamin and mineral supplement needs in normal children in the United States." *Pediatrics*, vol. 66. no. 6, December 1980, pp. 1015–20.

Pediatric Nutrition Handbook. AAP Publications, Evanston, Ill., 1979.

American Academy of Pediatrics News Bulletin. "Nutrition: special needs are outlined." Vol. 17, no. 2, Spring 1981, p. 15.

Anderson, N. G., et al. *Journal of the American Medical Association*, "The human protein index," vol. 246, no. 22, 4 December 1981, pp. 2620–2621.

Balli, F., ed. *Nutritional problems in childhood: proceedings of the international symposium.* Padua: Piccin Medical Books, 1978.

Barnett, H. L., ed. *Pediatrics.* 15th rev. ed. New York: Appleton-Century-Crofts, a public. div. of Prentice-Hall, Inc., 1972.

Barrett, D.E. "An approach to the conceptualization and assessment of social-emotional functioning in studying nutrition-behavior relationships." *The American Journal of Clinical Nutrition*, vol. 35, May 1982, pp. 1221–27.

Benedict, F.G., and Benedict, C. G. "The energy requirement of intense mental effort." *Science*, no. 71, 1930, 5 Suppl., p. 567.

Bond, J.T., et al, eds. *Infant and child feeding.* New York: Academic Press, 1981.

Brandt, I. "Brain growth, fetal malnutrition and clinical consequences." *Journal of Perinatal Medicine*, vol. 1 (1981), pp. 3–26.

Brazier, M.A.B., ed. *Growth and development of the brain: nutrition, genetics and environment.* New York: Raven Press, 1975.

RNA and brain function, memory and learning. Berkeley and Los Angeles: University of California Press, 1964.

British Medical Journal. "Nutrition and the brain." No. 6127, 17 June, 1978. pp. 1569–1570.

Canosa, C.A., ed. *Nutrition, growth and development: modern problems in paediatrics, vol. 14.* Basel, Switzerland: S. Karger, 1975.

Chernichovsky, D., and Coate, D. "The choice of diet for young children and its relation to children's growth." *The Journal of Human Resources,* vol. 15, no. 2, 1980, pp. 255–63.

Clarren, S.K. "Recognition of fetal alcohol syndrome." *Journal of the American Medical Association,* vol. 245, no. 23, 19 June, 1981, pp. 2436–2439.

Cone, T. E. Jr. *Two hundred years of feeding infants in America.* Columbus, Ohio: Ross Laboratories, 1976.

Cowan, W.M. "The development of the brain." *Scientific American,* September 1979, 241(3), pp. 113–33.

Cravioto, J., et al, eds. *Symposium on early malnutrition and mental development.* Stockholm: Almqvist and Wiksell, 1974.

Cummins, R. A., et al. "A developmental theory of environmental enrichment." *Science,* 12 August, 1977, pp. 692–694.

Dales, M. J. M. "Physicians divided on low-cholesterol diet for all." *Internal Medicine News,* vol. 15, no. 11, 1 June 1982, p. 1.

Dansky, K. H. "Assessing children's nutrition." *American Journal of Nursing,* October 1977, p. 1610.

Dobbing, J. "Human brain development and its vulnerability." *Indiana Medicine,* vol. 6, 1975, pp. 3–5.

Dobbing, J. "Maternal nutrition in pregnancy—eating for two?" Editorial in *Early Human Development,* vol. 5, 1981, pp. 113–115.

Dobbing, J., ed. *Maternal nutrition in pregnancy—eating for two?* Based on a workshop sponsored by Nestle Nutrition, Vaucluse, France. New York: Academic Press, 1981.

Dobbing, J., and Sands, J. "Comparative aspects of the brain growth spurt." *Early Human Development,* vol. 3, no. 1, 1979, pp. 79–83.

"Head circumference, biparietal diameter and brain growth in fetal and postnatal life." *Early Human Development,* vol. 2, no. 1, 1978, pp. 81–87.

Dobbing, J., and Sands, J. "Quantitative growth and development of the human brain." *Archives of Disease in Childhood*, vol. 48, 1973, pp. 757–767.

"Vulnerability of developing brain not explained by cell number/cell size hypothesis." *Early Human Development*, vol. 5 (1981), pp. 227–231.

Dodge, P., et al. *Nutrition and the developing nervous system.* St. Louis: C.V. Mosby Co., 1975.

Dwyer, J., et al. "Mental age and IQ of predominantly vegetarian children." *Journal of the American Dietetic Association*, vol. 76, February 1980, pp. 142–147.

Evans, D., et al. "Intellectual development and nutrition." *The Journal of Pediatrics*, vol. 97, no. 3, September 1980, pp. 358–363.

Ferchmin, P.A., and Eterovic, V.A. "Mechanism of brain growth by environmental stimulation." *Science*, August 1979, p. 522.

Filer, L.J. Jr. "Early nutrition: its long term role." *Hospital Practice*, vol. 13, no. 2, February 1978, pp. 87–95.

Foman, S.J. "A pediatrician looks at early nutrition." *Bulletin of the New York Academy of Medicine*, vol. 47, 1971, p. 569.

Foman, S.J. *Infant Nutrition.* 2nd ed. Philadelphia: Saunders and Co., 1974.

Foman, S.J., et al. "Recommendations for feeding normal infants." *Pediatrics*, vol. 63, no. 1, January 1979, pp. 52–59.

Freeman, H.E., et al. "Relations between nutrition and cognition in rural Guatemala." *American Journal of Public Health*, vol. 67, no. 3, March 1977, pp. 233–239.

Garry, P.J., ed., "Human nutrition, clinical and biochemical aspects." Washington, D.C.: The American Association for Clinical Chemistry, 1981.

Gerber Products Co. "Foods for Baby and Mealtime Psychology." Fremont, Michigan, rev. 4/72.

Gourlay, N. "Heredity versus environment: an integrative analysis." *Psychological Bulletin*, vol. 86. no. 3, 1979, pp. 596–615.

Hagerty, M. "Don't forget the iron." *The Boston Globe*, 14 October 1981.

Haire, D. "Instructions for nursing your baby." Pamphlet,

1969, from International Childbirth Education Association, P/D Center, P.O. Box 2728, Ridgemont Branch, Rochester, New York, 14626.

Harper, A.E., et al. "Effects of ingestion of disproportionate amounts of amino acids." *Physiological Review*, vol. 50: No. 3, July, 1970, pp. 428-558.

H. J. Heinz Co. "Heinz Baby Food ingredient listing." 1974. "How to read a Heinz Baby Food label." 1974.

Hirsch, J. "The interactions of nutrition and behavior." *The American Journal of Clinical Nutrition*, vol. 35, May 1982, pp. 1200-1.

Iversen, L.L. "The chemistry of the brain." *Scientific American*, September 1979, 241(3), pp. 134–149.

Jelliffe, D., and Jelliffe, E.F.P., eds. *Nutrition and growth*. New York: Plenum Press, 1979.

Kallen, D.J., ed. "Nutrition, development and social behavior." From *Proceedings of the conference on the assessment of tests of behavior from studies of nutrition in the Western Hemisphere*. U.S. Government Printing Office, DHEW, publication no. (NIH) 1973, pp. 73–242.

Kemberling, S.R. "Supporting breast feeding." *Pediatrics*, vol. 63, no. 1, January, 1979, pp. 60–63.

La Cerva, V.A. *Breastfeeding, a manual for health professionals*. Garden City, New York: Medical Examination Publication Co., Inc., 1981.

Lanzkowsky, P. "Iron deficiency, a public health problem." *Number One: Hematological Diseases in Children*, Mead Johnson Laboratories, p–120, 4/75, pp. 1–34.

Lawrence, R.A. *Breast feeding, a guide for the medical profession*. St. Louis: C.V. Mosby Co., 1980.

Leibel, R.L., et al. "Studies regarding the impact of micronutrient status on behavior in man: iron deficiency as a model." *The American Journal of Clinical Nutrition*, vol. 35, May 1982, 5 Suppl., pp. 1211–1221.

Lien, N.M., et al. "Early malnutrition and 'late' adoption: a study of their effects on the development of Korean orphans adopted into American families." *The American Journal of Clinical Nutrition*, vol. 30, October 1977, pp 1734–1739.

Lind, T. "Nutrient requirements during pregnancy—1." *The*

American Journal of Clinical Nutrition, supplement, vol. 34, no. 4, April 1981, pp. 669–678.

Mayer, J. *A diet for living.* New York: David McKay Co., Inc., 1975.

Mead Johnson Laboratories. "Why children don't eat and what to do about it." Literature no. 52, April 1971.

MD. "Food: man's lifelong fascination." Vol. 26, no. 8, July 1982, p. 138.

Morriss, F.H. Jr. "Placental factors conditioning fetal nutrition and growth." *The American Journal of Clinical Nutrition,* supplement, vol. 34, no. 4, April 1981, pp. 760–768.

McDonald, L. *Baby's recipe book.* Cranbury, New Jersey: A.S. Barnes and Co., Inc., 1972.

McLaren, D.S., and Burman, D., eds. *Textbook of Paediatric Nutrition.* 2nd ed. New York: Churchill Livingstone Co., 1982.

Merritt, D.H., ed. *Infant nutrition.* New York: Halstead Press, a div. of John Wiley and Sons Inc., 1976.

Moghissi, K.S., and Evans, T.N. *Nutritional impacts on women throughout life with emphasis on reproduction.* Hagerstown, Maryland: Harper and Row, 1977.

Naunton, E. "Don't want to take pills?" Knight-Ridder Service, *The Boston Globe,* 21 October 1981.

Nauta, W.J.H., and Feirtag, M. "The organization of the brain." *Scientific American,* September 1979, 241(3), pp. 88–111.

Palma, P.A., and Adcock, E.W. "Human milk and breast feeding." *AFP,* vol. 24, no. 1, pp. 173–181.

Passingham, R.E. "Brain size and intelligence in man." *Brain Behavior Evolution,* vol. 16, 1979, pp. 253–270.

Pediatric News. "Breast milk speeds head growth in tiny infants." Vol. 15, no. 4, April 1981, p. 30.

Pennington, J.A.T., and Church, H.N. *Bowes and Church's food values of portions commonly used.* 13th ed. Philadelphia: J.B. Lippincott Co., 1980.

Perkins, S.A. "Malnutrition and mental development." *Exceptional Children,* January 1977, pp. 214–219.

Physicians Washington Report. "Emotional growth linked to children's diet." Vol. 3, no. 9, October 1981.

Pipes, P. *Nutrition in infancy and childhood.* St. Louis: C.V. Mosby Co., 1977.

Reinis, S., and Goldman, J.M. *The development of the brain, biological and functional perspectives.* Springfield, Ill.: Charles C. Thomas, 1980.

Restack, R.M. *The brain—the last frontier.* Garden City, New York: Doubleday and Co., 1979.

Roberts, D.F., and Thomson, A.M., eds. *The biology of human fetal growth,* vol. 15, New York: Halstead Press, 1976.

Ross Laboratories. "McGill, Mitchell, Lauer on developmental nutrition: atherosclerosis." No. 9, 63604/March 1974.

"Similac with whey." Columbus, Ohio, D 507, July 1982.

Rush, D., et al. "Controlled trial of prenatal nutrition supplement defended." (Letter to the editor.) *Pediatrics,* vol. 66, no. 4, October 1980, pp. 656–658.

Rush, D., et al, eds. "Diet in pregnancy: a randomized controlled trial of nutritional supplements." March of Dimes Birth Defects Foundation, Birth Defects: Original article series, vol. 16, no. 3, New York: Alan R. Liss, 1980.

Sanders, T.A.B., et al. "Polyunsaturated fatty acids and the brain." (Letter to the editor.) *The Lancet,* 2 April 1977, pp. 751–752.

Schwartz, G.R. *Food power—how foods can change your mind, your personality and your life.* McGraw-Hill Co., 1979.

Scrimshaw, N.S., and Gordon, J.F., eds. *Proceedings of international conference on malnutrition, learning and behavior.* A symposium sponsored by the Nutrition Foundation Inc. and Massachusetts Institute of Technology. Cambridge: MIT Press, 1968.

Scriver, C.R. "Diets and genes: euphenic nutrition." *The New England Journal of Medicine,* vol. 297, no. 4, 28 July 1977, pp. 202–203.

Serban, G., ed. *Nutrition and mental functions.* New York: Plenum Press, 1975.

Slattery, J.S. "Nutrition for the normal healthy infant." *Maternal-Child Nursing,* March–April 1977, pp. 105–112.

Solomon, N. "No cow's milk before baby's a year old." *The Boston Globe,* Tuesday, 3 August 1981.

Stein, Z. "Nutrition and mental performance." *Science,* vol. 178, no. 4061, 10 November 1972, pp. 708–713.

Stoch, M.B., and Smythe, P.M. "Does undernutrition during infancy inhibit brain growth and subsequent intellectual development?" *Archives of Diseases in Childhood,* vol. 38, 1963, pp. 546–552.

The American Journal of Clinical Nutrition, vol. 34, April 1981, entire journal issue.

The Children's Hospital Medical Center, Boston, Massachusetts. "Diet recommendations for the '6 Food Groups' " 13011–5 c–12/71.

The Lancet, "Nutrition in critical periods of development." 30 July 1977, pp. 229–230.

Tsang, R.C., and Nichols Jr., B.L., eds. *Nutrition and child health, perspectives for the 1980's.* New York: Alan R. Liss, Inc., 1980.

United States Department Health Education and Welfare, Office of Child Development. "Your child from one to three." Children's Bureau public. No. 413-1964, reprinted 1971.

"Your child from three to four." Children's Bureau public. no. 446-1967, reprinted 1972.

Waletzky, L.R., ed. "Symposium on human lactation." U.S. Dept. HEW, public. no. (HSA) 79–5107, October, 1976.

Winick, M., and Brasel, J.A. "Early malnutrition and subsequent brain development." *Annals New York Academy of Sciences,* vol. 30, 30 November 1977, pp. 280–282.

Winick, M. "Early malnutrition, brain structure and function." Guest editorial in *Preventive Medicine,* 1977, pp. 358–360.

"Malnutrition and brain development." *The Journal of Pediatrics,* vol. 74, no. 5, May 1969, pp. 667–679.

"Nutrition." Guest editorial in *Pediatric Annals,* vol. 10, no. 11, November 1981.

Winick, M., ed. *Nutrition and development.* New York: John Wiley and Sons Inc., 1972.

Winick, M. "Nutrition and mental development." *Medical Clinics of North America,* vol. 54, no. 6, November 1970, pp. 1413–1429.

Winick, M., ed. *Nutrition pre- and postnatal development.* Vol. 1 of *Human nutrition—a comprehensive treatis.* New York: Plenum Press, 1979.

Winick, M. "Should you really be eating for two?" *Redbook,* January 1982.

Winick, M., and Rosso, P. "Head circumference and cellular

growth of the brain in normal and marasmic children."
The Journal of Pediatrics, vol. 74, no. 5, May 1969, pp.
774–778.

Wood, C.B.S., and Walker-Smith, J.A. *MacKeith's infant feeding
and feeding difficulties*. 6th ed. New York: Churchill Livingstone Co., 1981.

Young, C., et al. "Metabolic effects of meal frequency on normal young men." *Journal of the American Dietetic Association*, vol. 61, October 1972, pp. 391–398.

Yusuf, H.K.M., et al. "Cholesterol esters of the human brain
during fetal and early postnatal development: content
and fatty acid composition." *Journal of Neurochemistry*,
vol. 36, no. 2, 1981, pp. 707–714.

Zeskind, P.S., and Ramey, C.T. "Preventing intellectual and
interactional sequalae of fetal malnutrition: a longitudinal transactional and synergistic approach to development." *Child Development*, vol. 52, 1981, pp. 213–218.

INDEX

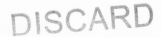